BIG FAT LIES

DAVID GILLESPIE is a recovering corporate lawyer, co-founder of a successful software company and consultant to the IT industry. He is also the father of six young children (including one set of twins). With such a lot of extra time on his hands, and 40 extra kilos on his waistline, he set out to investigate why he, like so many in his generation, was fat. He deciphered the latest medical findings on diet and weight gain and what he found was chilling. Being fat was the least of his problems. He needed to stop poisoning himself.

His books *Sweet Poison* and *The Sweet Poison Quit Plan* have a wide following, as do his Sweet Poison website and Raisin Hell blog.

sweetpoison.com.au

PRAISE FOR *THE SWEET POISON QUIT PLAN*

'For a "how to book", *The Sweet Poison Quit Plan* is actually a remarkably interesting read.' ANTHEA GLEESON, *TOOWOOMBA CHRONICLE*

'Gillespie's book is very readable and his quit plan has simple rules but detailed evidence.' *HOBART MERCURY*

PRAISE FOR *SWEET POISON*

'An eye-opening read on the health implications of too much sugar in our diet.' *GOOD HEALTH & MEDICINE*

'What's impressive about *Sweet Poison* is that Gillespie turns complex research on what happens to food inside our body and its relation to weight gain into a good read.' *SYDNEY MORNING HERALD*

'Comprehensive, thought-provoking and highly readable.' *THE AGE*

'David Gillespie's groundbreaking book on the dangers of a high sugar intake could well revolutionise the way you diet.' *A CURRENT AFFAIR*

'*Sweet Poison* is a worthy and impassioned effort by an Australian dad to share his surprising discoveries with struggling dieters and provoke further debate about the obesity epidemic.'
AUSTRALIAN BOOKSELLER & PUBLISHER

'I've lost 11 kg without being on a diet. It's good to know this book is non-fiction.' STEVE IRONS MP, MEMBER OF THE PARLIAMENTARY INQUIRY INTO OBESITY

BIG FAT LIES

HOW THE DIET INDUSTRY IS MAKING YOU SICK, FAT AND POOR

DAVID GILLESPIE

VIKING
an imprint of
PENGUIN BOOKS

For Lizzie, Anthony, James, Gwendolen,
Adam, Elizabeth and Finlayson.

VIKING

Published by the Penguin Group
Penguin Group (Australia)
250 Camberwell Road, Camberwell, Victoria 3124, Australia
(a division of Pearson Australia Group Pty Ltd)
Penguin Group (USA) Inc.
375 Hudson Street, New York, New York 10014, USA
Penguin Group (Canada)
90 Eglinton Avenue East, Suite 700, Toronto, Canada ON M4P 2Y3
(a division of Pearson Penguin Canada Inc.)
Penguin Books Ltd
80 Strand, London WC2R 0RL England
Penguin Ireland
25 St Stephen's Green, Dublin 2, Ireland
(a division of Penguin Books Ltd)
Penguin Books India Pvt Ltd
11 Community Centre, Panchsheel Park, New Delhi – 110 017, India
Penguin Group (NZ)
67 Apollo Drive, Rosedale, North Shore 0632, New Zealand
(a division of Pearson New Zealand Ltd)
Penguin Books (South Africa) (Pty) Ltd
24 Sturdee Avenue, Rosebank, Johannesburg 2196, South Africa

Penguin Books Ltd, Registered Offices: 80 Strand, London, WC2R 0RL, England

First published by Penguin Group (Australia), 2012

1 3 5 7 9 10 8 6 4 2

Text copyright © David Gillespie 2012

The moral right of the author has been asserted

Cover design by Daniel New © Penguin Group (Australia)
Text design by Evi Oetomo © Penguin Group (Australia)
Typeset in 11.5/17 pt Berkeley by Post Pre-press Group, Brisbane, Queensland
Printed and bound in Australia by McPherson's Printing Group, Maryborough, Victoria

National Library of Australia
Cataloguing-in-Publication data:

Gillespie, David, 1966–
Big fat lies: how the diet industry is making you sick, fat and poor / David Gillespie.

9780670076024 (pbk.)
Includes index.

Sugar – Health aspects.
Unsaturated fatty acids in human nutrition.
Weight loss – Health aspects.
Reducing diets.

613.28

penguin.com.au

CONTENTS

Introduction   1

**PART 1: The things we do that make no difference to
         our health**

1. Why diets don't work   11
2. The weight-loss methods we try   21
3. Exercise won't help you lose weight, either   41
4. Vitamins – don't waste your money   50
5. Salt and other minerals   85

PART 2: The real culprits: sugar and polyunsaturated fat

Introduction   101
6. Why we really gain weight – sugar   103
7. All about fats   123
8. Good fat, (very) bad fat   131
9. Polyunsaturated fats cause heart disease –
   and cholesterol doesn't   162
10. Polyunsaturated fats cause cancer   185

**PART 3: A practical guide to avoiding sugar and
         polyunsaturated fats**

Introduction   199
11. Cutting out sugar – or, more precisely, fructose   202
12. Cutting out polyunsaturated fats (specifically
    seed oils)   221
13. So what are we allowed to eat?   231

Epilogue   239
Notes   244
Acknowledgements   258
Index   261

Introduction

Diets and exercise won't help us lose weight. Vitamins and minerals are a waste of money and sometimes downright dangerous. Sugar makes us fat and sick. And polyunsaturated fat gives us cancer and works with sugar to give us heart disease. The evidence for all of these statements is abundant and unequivocal, but you won't hear anyone in the food and diet industries tell you so. If they did it would have an immediate impact on their sales, and when it comes to a choice between their money and your health, three guesses (oh, okay – one, then) which of these wins.

The sad truth is that people like you and me are uniquely vulnerable in a world of chronic disease caused by 'improvements' to our food supply. A choice between corporate profit today and your health in three decades is no choice to a drug or food company or their shareholders. A choice between a government bureaucrat staying 'on message' with what they've said for the last four decades and your future health is no choice to them if they want to keep their job. A choice between a charity (such as the Australian Heart

Foundation) attacking the source of its corporate sponsorship and how well you might be in 2041 is no choice to the people whose jobs depend on that sponsorship.

Even your doctor, the one person paid to have your health uppermost in their mind, is protecting you with both hands tied behind their back. At least one new medical journal article appears every 26 seconds. Just to keep up, your doctor would need to read 3300 journal articles a day (and that's before they started on the backlog). Obviously, even the most studious and dedicated doctor is doing nothing of the sort – doctors report spending about four hours a week reading journals, which is still a fair bit of time. This means they rely on the same sources of information (only with more detail) as the rest of us: drug companies, food manufacturers, charities and government employees.

This is a book about truth. I'm not a nutritionist or a doctor. I don't have a diet or a magic food to sell you. I'm just a lawyer who's worried about my health and the health of my family and who has a lot of time on his hands. This book exists only because I want you to know what the evidence actually says. Lawyers are trained in only one useful thing – evidence. This book sets out the evidence about our food. That evidence could not be more clear-cut, and what to do about it could not be more obvious.

I've chosen to lay out this evidence in a book because books are the only form of mass media available to me that are not influenced by advertising. The companies that benefit from our continued consumption of sugar, polyunsaturated vegetable oils, statin drugs, vitamins and diet plans spend more on advertising (by a country mile) than all other businesses combined. A book it must be – there's no other way to communicate in detail the information it contains without the story being influenced by someone whose job depends on advertising.

What can we do?

Apart from this book, you don't need to buy anything. You just need to stop consuming foods containing two substances introduced into our diets in the 1850s – sugar and polyunsaturated vegetable oils – and avoid the 'cures' introduced after World War II. The inconvenient fact is that this means eliminating almost all processed foods from your diet.

The good news, however, is that saving yourself from the insidious damage being done by sugar and polyunsaturated vegetable oils is as simple as knowing what you're eating. The even better news is that it will cost you nothing. You don't need to pay a diet guru to become thin. You don't need to subsist on a diet of Tibetan cantaloupes infused with dolphin tears. You don't need to pay a muscle-bound fitness fanatic to abuse you in a public park. And you don't need to go to weekly meetings for a dose of group humiliation. By doing nothing apart from avoiding two ingredients, you'll lose weight, skip past a list of chronic diseases you couldn't jump over (even if you were being yelled at by a lycra-clad trainer) and save yourself a bucket of money while you're at it.

Our food supply

It might seem like our supermarkets are full of newfangled products that weren't there a week ago, let alone last century, but when we brush aside the marketing, very little has changed about our food supply in thousands of years. We're still mammals that require carbohydrates and some fats for fuel. And we still need protein to make our muscles and other bits. They can dress it up in a pretty box and claim it's new or better or healthier than it was last week, but our bodies have very simple food requirements. Our metabolism can't read labels and our biochemistry is what it is, no matter what a marketer might tell us.

There have, however, been two very important changes to our food supply in the last hundred years. These changes weren't introduced to make us healthier or better people, but for two very simple commercial reasons: increased sales and lower costs. Commercial quantities of sugar were added to food because food with sugar sells better than food without sugar (yes, it really is that simple). And man-made fats were introduced because foods made with polyunsaturated seed oils are cheaper than foods made with animal fats. This means, of course, that there are powerful financial incentives to keep both in the food supply for as long as possible.

Why sugar and polyunsaturated fats are bad for us

In my books *Sweet Poison* and *The Sweet Poison Quit Plan* I went through the evidence against sugar in detail. When I first started to look into things, I was motivated by a very simple plan – to be less fat. And it worked. But along the way I discovered that science says much more about sugar than that it induces a fat tummy. In fact, sugar bypasses delicately balanced systems that tightly control our appetite and blood-sugar levels. Once our system is out of balance, we career like an out-of-control car towards the cliff face of obesity and a list of other chronic diseases that grows with the publication of each new study. Oh, and just for fun, sugar is highly addictive and therefore impossible to eliminate from our diet without conscious effort.

As I read the evidence against sugar, I kept coming across studies on fat. It was clear that fat could not possibly do the things the nutrition dogma suggested. It was also abundantly clear that once we fix the appetite-control system broken by sugar, fat will take care of itself. Once we're back in possession of a functional appetite-control system, we can and do tightly regulate our fat consumption automatically. But under the surface of the studies I read was a worrying line of evidence that suggested it matters very much what type of fat we consume, because although our body can't detect whether fats are saturated or unsaturated, these fats can still make a dramatic difference to how our body functions.

Strange as it sounds, to most cells in our body, oxygen is a dangerous substance. Oxygen is highly reactive. When it reacts with iron we get rust. When it reacts with wood, we get fire (if the temperature is right). And when it reacts with fat, it breaks that fat down into a range of dangerous chemicals and destroys the integrity of any cell made from fat – which is every cell in our body. We have two defences against this process of oxidation. First, most of the fat we make (and until a hundred years ago, most of the fat we ate) does not oxidise much – saturated fat is the stainless steel of the cellular world. Secondly, for any fat that *is* oxidised, we have our own little fire brigade – a bunch of homemade chemicals called anti-oxidants.

Polyunsaturated fats are exactly the opposite: they react quickly with oxygen. This is a very, very bad thing in a body that needs to be as oxygen-resistant as possible. Oxidated fats can lead to the random destruction and out-of-control cellular growth otherwise known as cancer. And they can create the lesions that lead to heart disease. Both processes are helped enormously by the huge quantities of sugar in a normal Western diet. In the last hundred years we've gradually and systematically replaced all the saturated fats in our diet with destructive polyunsaturated fats. And just for good measure, we've added huge quantities of sugar to make the destruction happen quickly.

Sugar has given us diabetes, dementia and obesity. And polyunsaturated fats have given us cancer. Together they've combined to give us heart disease. Both were added to our diets in bulk long before ingredients were tested for their health impacts or safety. And both have combined to create seemingly untreatable epidemics in just three generations.

What's a seed oil?

We've been told that the secret to curing heart disease is to consume unsaturated vegetable oils rather than saturated animal fats. So now all the fats in our processed foods are labelled 'vegetable oil' and the labels are rarely more specific than that.

The irony is that there is no such thing as oil from a vegetable. The products being pushed to us as vegetable oils are fruit oils (coconut, palm, olive or avocado), nut oils (macadamia, peanut, pecan, and so on) or seed oils (canola, sunflower, soy or rice bran).

There's nothing much wrong with the fruit oils (I'll go into why later) and some of the nut oils are okay, too. But the seed oils are extraordinarily dangerous. And unfortunately they make up almost all of the 'vegetable oils' in our food.

The diet, exercise and supplements industries

Cashing in on the confusion and misinformation about the causes of obesity, heart disease and cancer, a group of huge industries has come of age. The diet, exercise and supplements industries did not exist before World War II, but in 60 short years they've built an empire that rivals those of sugar and seed oils themselves. At first the sugar and seed-oil sellers were happy to encourage these growing healthy-living sectors – after all, they made sure everybody was looking in exactly the wrong direction – but now the sugar and seed-oil mega-corporations are scooping up those sectors, too.

There's never been any evidence that counting calories (or fat or carbs) will make us thin. The evidence has never suggested that exercise will have any effect on our weight other than to increase our appetite. Nor has it given credence to the theory that we're functionally deficient in any of the substances in a multivitamin tablet or any other supplement. But this complete lack of evidence has not slowed the exponential growth of the diet, exercise and supplements industries. And just like desperate gamblers, we keep coming back to them, despite abundant proof that it will fail just as it did last time.

About this book

This book lays out the evidence against sugar and seed oils, and provides practical and effective advice on how to avoid eating them. The first part of this book gives the facts about the things we're urged to do every minute of our waking lives. It tells us why diets will not make us thin, why exercise makes us hungrier rather than lighter and why supplements are just a very effective way to flush your hard-earned dosh away. The second part of the book presents the evidence against the real culprits of chronic disease: sugar and seed oils. And the third part translates that evidence into practical advice on how to live in a society where almost every man-made food is filled to the brim with sugar and seed oils.

The first two parts do occasionally dive deeply into the evidence. I try to translate it into language even I could understand, but it does get hairy at times, so stick with me – it's worth it. In this book I attack most of the basic assumptions we make about our health. I don't do that lightly. It's important that the evidence be presented in full for two reasons. First, vested interests and their handmaidens will attack what I say repeatedly, so I must present the evidence clearly and unequivocally. Secondly, I don't expect you to trust me any more than I trust the folks selling us fructose, seed oils, statins and weight-loss programs. You must be able to jump past my interpretation and go straight to the source (if you want to). The comprehensive 'Notes' section at the back of this book gives details of the original scientific papers and books from which the information in this book is drawn.

Commercial forces have provided us with the most perfectly destructive combination of chronically dangerous chemicals I could imagine. And those same commercial forces have worked to ensure we do nothing effective about changing that. This book exists because I desperately hope that with a little knowledge we can all vote with our feet and change the rules of the game before the game kills us.

Strap yourself in – let's do this thing.

PART 1

THE THINGS WE DO
THAT MAKE NO DIFFERENCE
TO OUR HEALTH

1. WHY DIETS DON'T WORK

We're fat because we eat too much. To be more precise, we're fat because we consume more energy than we expend. The key to not being fat, according to those who think they should tell us what to do about it, is either to exercise some willpower and eat less or just to exercise or, preferably, both. This advice is based on the first law of thermodynamics. It says that energy cannot be created or destroyed, merely changed from one form to another. It's a law about physical forces, particularly heat and mechanical energy. In the nutrition and diet industry, however, it's usually rendered more like 'energy in must equal energy out' or just called 'the energy-balance equation'. Sometimes they'll even write an actual equation (I guess to make it look more scientific):

weight gain (energy balance) = energy in (food) − energy out (exercise)

The first law of thermodynamics has been hijacked by nutritionists because it sounds a bit like it should apply to dieting. As a result, it's used more today in human nutrition than in any other domain of human endeavour. The first law is quoted with any information on diet products, exercise or weight-loss programs. And the government throws it in our face almost as regularly. We're told that the only way we can lose weight is either to consume less energy (fewer calories) or burn more energy by exercising.

What's a calorie?

Food energy is measured in calories. One calorie is the amount of energy required to increase the temperature of 1 gram of water by 1 degree Celsius. To heat enough water for a cup of coffee from room temperature to boiling point would take about 20 000 calories of energy.

A calorie is therefore a very small unit of measurement, so dietitians often abbreviate kilocalories (thousands of calories) to 'Calories' (with a capital 'C') as a sort of shorthand. Heating the cup of coffee would actually take just 20 Calories in the sense most people understand, as used in food labelling.

The metric equivalent of the calorie is the joule. Scientifically speaking, one small 'c' calorie is equivalent to 4.185 joules and one capital 'C' Calorie equals 4.185 *kilo*joules (kJ). Throughout this book I've used calorie in lower case to mean the equivalent of 4.185 kilojoules.

Counting calories

Most food contains 4 calories of energy per gram. The exceptions are fat, which has 9 calories per gram, and alcohol, which has 7. So if the calorie content of one serve of food is higher than that of another serve of similar weight, that's really just another way of saying that one has more fat than the other (or more booze, but let's stay out of the bottle shop for now).

Because fat has more than twice the calories per gram of protein or carbohydrate, it's often the target of calorie-restriction marketing from the food and diet industries. And it's one reason the Australian Government tells us to limit our fat intake (the other being heart disease – for more on this, see below).

Gram for gram, you can eat more than twice as much of a carbohydrate or protein and not unbalance your energy equation. Sounds logical, right? All we have to do if we want to lose weight is eat fewer calories. And as long as we keep eating fewer calories, the weight will just keep coming off. It's a simple, logical message, and that's why it has so much traction for people who want us to buy their diet products. The only problem is that the research on diets shows that it's utter nonsense.

If we're getting fat by misjudging the number of calories we shove in our gob, then we're doing some pretty extraordinary maths every time we open our mouths. Think about what you ate and drank yesterday. I bet if you thought about it for a few minutes you could come up with a pretty thorough list. Now tell me how many calories (or kilojoules, if you want to be all pernickety) that was. If you have the remotest clue what the answer is, you're doing better than me and probably just about everybody. Did you eat 2200 calories or was it 1800 or maybe 2723? Perhaps you kept a very detailed list, weighed everything, had a good calorie-counting book on hand and, after several hours pounding the calculator, concluded you consumed exactly 2143.28 calories. Now how about the day before yesterday? That's right, get out the scales, the calculator and the books again. What are the chances it was exactly 2143.28? How about the day before that? Let's face it, unless you're in solitary confinement and a bloke with a truncheon is weighing and dispensing the same food to you every day, the number of calories you eat is going to vary quite a bit from day to day.

Today you might have been running late and skipped your morning coffee (mine's a tall whole-milk latte, by the way, approximately 176 calories at Starbucks if the serving is exactly 355 ml). Or perhaps, in a coffee-deprived and weakened state, you were talked into 'having fries with that' at lunchtime (a medium serve of McDonald's fries has 368 calories if it weighs exactly 104 grams, not a fry more or less). Maybe you mowed the lawn and then had two brewskis to celebrate (135 calories per can or stubby). Clearly, the exact number of calories we consume in a day varies a lot based on what we're doing, what we feel like eating, who we're with and what else is going on in our life. It's also very clear that the only certainty is we won't eat exactly the same number of calories as we did yesterday or we will tomorrow.

A kilogram of body fat stores about 9000 calories. Most of us didn't wake up one day and find ourselves 20 kilograms overweight. It takes years of dedicated work. For most of us, it takes 10–20 years to add 20 kilograms (although the older we get, the easier it seems to be). To gain weight at the rate of 1 kilogram per year, traditional logic says we'd have to consume 9000 more calories than we needed in that year, about 25 calories extra a day, day in, day out, for 20 years (7300 days). That's one mouthful of a medium latte, maybe an eighth of a fry, perhaps just under a quarter of a Monte Carlo biscuit (and pretty much just reading the label on a packet of Tim Tams).

As ludicrous as it might seem, that's our margin for error. If we miscalculate our calorie requirements by a quarter of a Monte Carlo every day, we'll put on 20 kilograms in 20 years. Since most of us don't carry around a set of scales and have no idea what the calorie content of our food is, even if we did weigh it, nailing the exact number of calories to eat in a day (with a 25 calorie margin of error) is very daunting. Imagine how hard your pet dog or cat finds it, given they can't read, or operate the scales with their paws.

But that's exactly what health authorities want us to do. They tell us that one reason we're fat is that we eat too many calories. They tell us that this is a choice we make every time we put food in our mouth. If we just managed not to eat those extra 25 calories per day, they say, there'd be no obesity epidemic. To help us, they make food manufacturers and fast-food vendors prominently display how many calories (approximately) are in the food we eat. The theory appears to be that if we know there are 368 calories in a medium serve of fries, we'll add that to our running tally for the day and stop eating as soon as we reach the magic recommended daily calorie intake (which varies according to gender, age, ethnicity and activity level, and is not published anywhere we're likely to find it).

I have no idea how many calories I ate yesterday and I certainly don't know whether it was 25 calories more or less than the day before. Clearly no one (unless they have an eating disorder) is actually weighing everything they eat and drink and fretting over those extra 25 calories. Clearly most of us never think about the number of calories we eat and, even if we did, we have neither the skills nor the information to avoid a 25 calorie mistake every day. But when a health authority tells us we're fat because we eat too many calories, they're also telling us we have to eliminate those 25 extra calories a day. In other words, we must *consciously* reduce – by a micro-shade – the amount of something that's highly variable and completely unknown. Okay, you might be thinking, I don't know how many calories I'm eating, but when I'm dieting, I do try to eat lower calorie foods – surely that knocks off the 25 calories (and many more)? Well, yes, but that's assuming your body doesn't compensate for the lack of calories. And the bad news is, the research says that's exactly what the body does.

How our bodies react to calorie restriction

There haven't been many times in medical history when research-ers have been permitted to starve humans on purpose. But in the dying days of World War II, one of the founding fathers of human nutrition in America, Ancel Keys (much more on him later, in Chapter 8), was given the go-ahead to study the effects of starva-tion on human volunteers. He recruited 36 healthy young men of normal weight from the ranks of conscientious objectors to the military draft.

The men were accommodated in the football stadium of the University of Minnesota and starved for 24 weeks. Depending on their initial weight, they were restricted to consuming between 1600 and 1800 calories a day while still working and performing physical exercise – they had to walk 15 kilometres a week. The pur-pose of the experiment was to simulate the starvation that would be occuring in war-torn Europe. The researchers would then refeed the men according to different schedules so that the US had real data on the best diet for the recovery of Europe.

As expected, the men experienced significant weight loss (25 per cent on average). Their diet was strictly controlled, so it makes sense that if they were fed a lot less than they needed, their body had to compensate. It did so by dropping muscle and fat mass. What was less expected were their other symptoms. The men immediately lost all sex drive. They were constantly hungry, became tired and lethargic and slept as much as they were allowed. They reported feeling cold all the time and struggled even to lift their feet over the gutter when crossing the road. Eventually, the researchers noted that their subjects developed significant apathy, irritability, loss of cognitive function (not thinking clearly) and depression.

And just in case you have an aversion to olden-time research, much more modern data are now becoming available. Medical researchers aren't allowed to starve people on purpose nowadays, but that doesn't stop them studying people who've been purposely starved for less high-minded purposes (oh, say, for a television show). Researchers from the Pennington Biomedical Research Center in Baton Rouge accompanied *Biggest Loser* participants on set in the US season 8 (2009). They presented their findings at a meeting of the Obesity Society in San Diego in 2010. As you might expect, they found that by Week 6, participants had lost 13 per cent of their body weight and by Week 30 it was 39 per cent. But the study revealed a much more interesting finding, with hard data to back it up.

As we lose weight our metabolism slows. We don't need to produce as much energy as quickly because we have less weight to carry around. So, just as a small car needs a smaller, more fuel-efficient engine than a large truck, we can run our engines at a lower, more fuel-efficient rate. But this study found that by Week 6, the contestants' metabolisms had slowed by 244 calories per day more than would have been expected from their weight loss alone. By Week 30, they were burning an astounding 504 calories per day less than expected. Effectively, that means they'd have to eat one meal less a day than someone who was naturally the same weight, just to maintain their weight loss. Perhaps that's why so few *Biggest Loser* contestants manage to keep the weight off.

Our body's response to insufficient calories is to demand more, a response we know as hunger. When calories aren't forthcoming, the body compensates by progressively shutting down energy-consuming systems and then using up muscle and fat. Physical movement is minimised, sleep is the preferred option, body temperature is lowered and eventually even thinking (cognitive function uses a massive 25 per cent of the energy we consume) is minimised. None of these actions is a conscious decision.

The Minnesota trial and *The Biggest Loser* are pretty extreme experiments, but there's nothing to suggest our bodies aren't up to this sort of caper all the time. Our body detects any reduction in available energy and compensates by lowering our peripheral (arm and leg) temperature, doing things a bit more slowly than it otherwise might or making us sleep for slightly longer than we usually would.

Intentionally reducing calories also assumes we don't accidentally compensate by eating more of something else. The men in the starvation experiment and the contestants on *The Biggest Loser* had no choice, but our body's first line of defence to intentional deprivation would be to ask for more food by making us feel hungry. Our ability to resist that signal varies enormously over time and depends a lot on our motivation and circumstances. When we ignore it, as we do with determination in the first few weeks of a diet, our body simply starts cutting down on energy consumption and, yes, losing weight (but not necessarily fat). But it will only do this for as long as we can resist our body's constant demand for food. Suggesting we can count calories makes the fundamentally flawed assumption that our body has a fixed calorie requirement and all we have to do is feed it less than that.

If the studies above demonstrate nothing else, they tell us that our caloric needs are a moving target that reacts to every action we take. But that reality still eludes those who decide nutrition policy in this country. Many Australian states have now enacted laws requiring fast-food manufacturers to tell us exactly how many calories are in the food we eat.

Do calorie labels work?

The Victorian plan is a straight copy of the calorie-labelling laws enacted in New York City in mid-2008. But a Yale and New York

University study showed that the effect of these laws was exactly nothing. The researchers interviewed customers at multiple restaurants of four fast-food chains (McDonald's, Wendy's, Burger King and KFC) and, to see what customers had ordered, collected 1156 receipts from them two weeks before the laws were introduced and four weeks afterwards. A similar population in a state without the law (just across the Hudson River in New Jersey) was used as the control. The locations were chosen because they both have a high proportion of obesity and diabetes among poor minority populations.

In New York and in the control city before the laws came into effect, the average customer ordered a meal of 825 calories. Afterwards, the New York customers had bumped their orders up to 846 calories but the control customers were still ordering the same as before. People ordered *more* calories *after* the signs were introduced. And while that's probably just a statistical anomaly, there's certainly no suggestion that the signs had any effect at all on what people ordered.

We don't measure food calories. We don't add them up. We don't record their day-to-day variation and we certainly can't manage them to within 25 calories per day. What we eat, when we eat and how many calories our food contains are all managed on autopilot. If we do more exercise we eat more. If we skip lunch, we eat more at dinner. We do this not because we've calculated the calorie content of our lunch (or read it on a fast-food menu) and compared it with our normal dinner, but because we're hungry. Sure, we can decide to skip a meal, but then we'll be missing energy the body was counting on, and the amount we eat at the next meal will be automatically adjusted.

The number of calories we eat is on a very finely balanced feedback loop. The total is constantly changing and there's no way we could consciously control our daily calorie intake to the precision of a few calories a day. If weight control really depended on that, then most of us would be on a constant rollercoaster, veering wildly from underweight to overweight and back again.

2. THE WEIGHT-LOSS METHODS WE TRY

Most (about two-thirds) of Australians weigh more than we should. And even if we didn't have the government and the weight-loss industry constantly pointing that out, we'd probably all like to lose more than a few kilos. A similar situation in the US explains of course why, at any given time, 45 per cent of American women and 30 per cent of US men admit they're trying to lose weight. If we throw in those who are just trying to maintain their weight with diets (in the US 35 per cent of both men and women), then I estimate that four out of five of us is currently on a diet (yes you are, go on, admit it). It should come as no great surprise, then, that a huge industry has developed around helping us lose that weight.

In the 2010/11 financial year, Australians spent almost $800 million on diet programs, diet foods and weight-loss surgery. But that's the mere tip of the iceberg. Before we sign up for Jenny Craig or Weight Watchers we usually do quite a bit of DIY. We skip meals, limit portion sizes, count calories, limit fat intake (usually by eating food labelled 'diet' or 'lite') or try to exercise a bit more.

All commercial diets require us to deprive ourselves of a major food group. The calorie-counters want us to cut our fat intake to less than 25 per cent of our total intake and the low-carbers want us to do something similar or even more extreme with carbohydrates. Low-carbers initially have an easier time of it because the carbohydrate-driven hunger signal is shut down, but in the end the research says that all diets get to the same place. They don't work. Or, to be more accurate, they do work for a little while, but they never result in long-term (two years or more) weight loss.

And if you think about it, that must be right. If any diet actually did work, pure economics would take over. The diet that worked would be inundated with obese participants. Out the other end they'd all come, newly slimmed down, and become walking advertisements for the fabulous diet. No other diet would stand a chance in the market, and pretty soon the diet that worked would be the only show in town. But that's not what happens. Each year there are more diets on the market than the year before, and not one of them seems to be able to produce enough satisfied customers to put an end to the diet industry.

With the exception of surgery (and I'll come to that), all dietary weight-loss approaches, both commercial and homemade, share two common themes. They require us to exercise our willpower (well, suffer, really – if you ain't suffering, it ain't a diet) and reduce the number of calories we consume. None of them is any more sophisticated than that. The dietary methods used to limit calorie intake can be divided into three main camps: low-fat/low-calorie, meal-replacers and low-carb.

The basic food groups

Our food can be divided into three primary groups:

1. **Carbohydrates**, which largely make up edible plant and seed material, such as fruits, vegetables, grains and sugars. Since we're not that close to the land these days, you'll recognise carbohydrate foods as the more highly processed breads, biscuits and breakfast cereals. Carbohydrates are made by plants converting the energy from sunlight into stored sugars.

2. **Proteins**, of which our most abundant source is meat. Animals (including us) eat carbohydrates for energy and use that energy to build proteins, largely in the form of muscle. Of course carnivores and omnivores (like us) can circumvent the whole plant-to-muscle process simply by eating another animal and stealing its proteins.

3. **Fats**, which are energy-storage molecules used by plants (oils) and animals (fats). Fats don't contain water, so they can store more than twice as much energy as an equivalent amount of carbohydrate or protein. Fats are a great shortcut to energy for an animal that hasn't eaten for a while. Just suck down some fat and you'll have instant energy.

Low-fat/low-calorie diets

The fat-watchers have noticed that gram for gram, fat (9 calories per gram) has more than twice as many calories as carbohydrate or protein (both 4 calories per gram). A kilo of fat (whether it's on the table or on our bottom) stores about 9000 calories of energy, so calorie-watchers base their diets on the elimination of fat calories. If we need 2300 calories per day to run our body (a fairly typical amount for an adult woman), then feeding us, say, 1300 calories per day will result in an 'energy deficit' of 1000 calories per day and this will ultimately add up to the 9000 calories per kilo we need to lose. Following that maths through, it would take about nine days per kilo lost (or about a year to lose 40 kilos).

The fat-watcher theory appears to be that we measure how much we eat with our eyes rather than our appetite. Because carbohydrates (such as sugar) have less than half the calories of fat, a clever food manufacturer can make a low-fat meal that looks exactly the same as its full-fat brother, simply by increasing the carbs (usually sugar) and lowering the fats. The theory goes that because we can't see calories but we can see food, we'll lose weight if we substitute lower calorie carbohydrates for higher calorie fats. That means we could eat 50 per cent more no-fat yoghurt (114 calories in a 200 gram serve) than full-fat yoghurt (168 calories per 200 grams). There's a reason that sounds just a bit familiar. Three of the most popular Australian examples of this approach are Weight Watchers, Lite n' Easy and Jenny Craig (now owned by Nestlé).

Weight Watchers

Weight Watchers enforces its low-fat regime by using a point system. The prospective Weight Watcher is given a point target, which aims to create a 1000 calorie deficit a day so that they lose 1 kilogram every nine days. The idea is that if the punter simply sticks to that point target (or less), then the weight will simply melt away. The points for individual foods are worked out using a complex and patented calculation that converts the calorie, fat and fibre content of any food into a number of points. The equations have recently been changed (see opposite); but it's still the case that the more fat in the food, the higher its Weight Watchers point value, and the less of it you're allowed to eat. Weight Watchers also requires its clients to attend weekly group sessions to ensure they stick to the plan.

The Weight Watchers formula

In November 2010, Weight Watchers changed its formula for calculating points. The old formula was driven by the calorie – and therefore fat – content of the food, with an allowance for fibre. It's top secret, but the Weight Watchers patent (yep, there's a patent – several, in fact) suggests it looked something like this:

1 point = (calories/50) + (fat in grams/12) – (dietary fibre in grams or 4, whichever is the smaller number)

In other words, 1 point is equal to the number of calories in a food serving divided by 50. The value increases by about one point for every 12 grams of fat, and drops by about 1 point for every 5 grams of fibre.

Food manufacturers who wanted to create foods for Weight Watchers could achieve a good point score either by bumping up the fibre content or dropping the fat content (usually by replacing it with sugar). This is one reason we've been inundated with high-fibre muffins and high-sugar muesli bars labelled as diet food.

The old formula paid no attention to the amount of protein or carbohydrate in a food, but the new ProPoints formula ('Pro' stands for protein, presumably), which is also top secret, supposedly addresses this issue. Based on the relevant patents, the formula looks a bit like this:

1 point = (16 x protein in grams + 19 x carbohydrate in grams + 45 x fat in grams) – (14 x fibre in grams), all divided by 175

The first part of the equation is pretty much the formula for calculating the calorie content of a food:

1 calorie = (16 x protein in grams + 16 x carbohydrate in grams + 36 x fat in grams) – (0 x fibre in grams), all divided by 4

Just as in the old Weight Watchers formula, fat and fibre are the big determinants in the new one, but at least it now recognises that carbohydrates such as sugar will be used as substitutes, and there's a very slight penalty for carbohydrates (19) versus protein (16).

A manufacturer that wanted to stay on the good side of this formula would choose to replace fat with protein rather than carbohydrate. The penalty (3/175 points per gram) is pretty small and there are big bonuses for fibre, so be on the lookout for the addition of loads of fibre-like sugars, such as inulin, instead.

Jenny Craig and Lite n' Easy

Being owned by the world's largest processed-food manufacturer, Nestlé, Jenny Craig takes a more direct approach. It cuts out the middleman and the points calculator and goes straight to supplying the low-fat food, with some one-on-one counselling. Lite n' Easy follows a similar model and even delivers the food to your house – but doesn't bother with the counselling. If the punter eats only what they're supposed to eat from the supplied foods (plus some allowances for fresh fruit and vegetables), they'll be eating a low-fat and therefore calorie-limited diet.

Weight Watchers, Jenny Craig and Lite n' Easy are all straightforward fat-elimination (calorie-counting) diets. Because the cost of the food isn't included in the Weight Watchers program, it often comes out looking less expensive than the other two in head-to-head comparisons.

Do low-fat diets actually work?

Weight Watchers and Jenny Craig are the two biggest commercial diet-providers in the world and both have recently been tested in randomised, controlled trials. In this kind of trial, the participants are randomly assigned either to a group following the diet or one not following the diet (the control group), and the progress of each group is directly measured against the other. Both trials compared the diet system being studied with what they called a 'self-help group'. The self-helpers were given information on losing weight and offered a follow-up counselling session with a dietitian, but otherwise left to their own devices.

Both studies were funded by the folks selling the respective diets, who also provided all the meals (for Jenny Craig) and counselling sessions (for both) free of charge. The group on Weight Watchers were provided with vouchers for free attendance at weekly Weight Watchers sessions in their area. This would normally have cost them $936 for the duration of the trial. The Jenny Craig group also had access to free weekly one-on-one counselling sessions with a Jenny Craig consultant. If they'd had to pay for all this luvin, it would have cost them $718 for the counselling and $6240 for the food. Because of all these factors, the studies are not completely real-world examples. In the real world, we're supposed to pay for the diet, not the other way around. Given that, these studies probably represent the best possible scenario in terms of keeping people motivated and sticking to the diet for the entire length of the study, which in each case was two years. Even so, 30 per cent of Weight Watchers and 9 per cent of Jenny Craig participants had dropped out by the end.

After two full years on either Weight Watchers or Jenny Craig, the participants enjoyed less than stellar results. The calories-in, calories-out theory suggests that if the rate of calorie deficiency was maintained for the whole two years, both groups should have lost about 1 kilogram every 10 days, which would have them weighing 72 kilograms less at the end than at the start. Obviously that didn't happen, because if it did, most of them would have weighed in at around the 21 kilogram mark. Here's what actually happened.

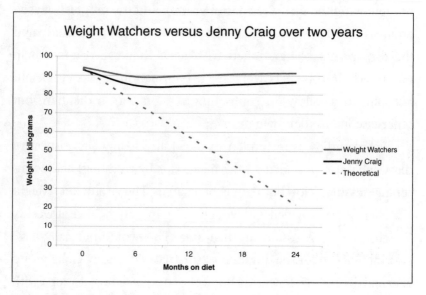

The Weight Watchers group started out weighing 94.2 kilograms on average and after two years of weekly meetings (including public weigh-ins, *Biggest Loser* style) and counting calories (sorry, points) they weighed on average 91.3 kilograms, an average weight loss of just 2.9 kilograms. But those average weights hide an even more depressing story. By the end, 37 per cent of those participants who finished the trial were the same weight or had *gained* weight instead of losing it. Other research indicates that we can assume the folks who left the trial early (one in three) did so because they were getting nowhere or putting on weight, which implies that more than half of the original participants went in the wrong direction. The participants were obese (defined in this trial as anything above 83 kilograms) at the start and two years later they were still obese.

The folks in the Jenny Craig study did a little better, but the free meals might have had a bit to do with it. They were provided with two free meals a day and an eating plan designed to ensure they ate 42–68 per cent of their normal calorie intake. But the results are still a long way short of the mathematically expected 72 kilogram weight loss. After two years of free Jenny Craig meals and weekly counselling, the average dieter managed to drop from 92.2 kilograms to 86.6 kilograms (which means they were still obese – in this trial defined as anything above 81 kilograms). Even the self-helpers managed to drop 2 kilograms! The good news is that if you can convince Jenny Craig to pay for your food and counselling (don't hold your breath), you can expect to lose about 6 kilograms in two years. If you started out obese, you'd still be obese and you'd have been starving for two whole years, but your pants might fit a little better.

Meal-replacement diets

Meal-replacers take calorie-counting to a whole new level. Fat-watchers usually try to eliminate enough calories to lose (theoretically) 0.5–1 kilo a week, which means cutting food intake by about 1000 calories a day. Meal-replacers want better results faster, so these kinds of diets aim for a cut of 1200 calories per day and some (often called very low-calorie diets or VLCDs) aim for a cut of 1500 calories per day.

The diets ask us to replace two (or if it's a VLCD, three) meals a day with a very low-calorie and therefore largely fat-free alternative. We're allowed to eat one meal, which can be anything we like as long as it's a small portion of lean meat and vegetables. The replacements are usually powdered milk drinks or shakes, but can sometimes be chocolate bars, soups or even breakfast cereal (see list below). The replacements can generally only be purchased from pharmacies and some only after a 'consultation' with a 'weight-loss professional' (and the payment of a fee), but very few pharmacies don't sell shakes of some description, with or without the consultation, and more and more such products are available in supermarkets, where the only consultation you're likely to get is the one asking you how you'd like to pay for it.

The best known meal-replacers are:

- Atkins Advantage
- Betty Baxter
- Celebrity Slim
- FatBlaster
- Herbalife
- Kate Morgan
- Kellogg's Special K Challenge
- Nestlé Optifast
- Optislim
- Rapid Loss
- Slim Right
- The Biggest Loser Club
- Tony Ferguson
- Ultraslim
- Vita Diet
- Xantrax
- Xndo.

The overwhelming majority of the replacements are milkshakes. The recipe varies a little between brands but the typical shake is one-third milk protein and almost half sugar, with just a smidgen of milk fat for taste (pretty much powdered milk plus sugar plus multi-vitamins). When mixed with water to reconstitute the powdered milk, one shake is intended to replace one meal, but there are precious few calories (only about 200) in them. This is about the same as a small (300 ml) chocolate milk and about a quarter of the calories an adult man would eat in a normal meal. The combined effect of replacing two meals a day with a shake would therefore be to halve the number of calories the average person would eat.

Meal-replacement diets often have stunning initial success because they massively restrict calories. If you can stick to the diet – and this will be difficult because the sweetener most of them use is fructose, which encourages the body to ratchet up the appetite – then having only a 200 calorie glass of sweetened milk for two (or even all) of your meals will probably knock off quite a bit of weight.

Does meal replacement actually work?

In 2005, the University of Pennsylvania School of Medicine reviewed the available evidence on meal-replacement diets. High-quality studies were not falling out of the trees. The best they could assemble were conducted by the diet vendors on folks who were completing the diets under the supervision of one of their 'wellness centres'. But on the basis of these studies, the researchers concluded that an obese person can expect to lose 15–25 per cent of their body weight in the first six months of 'treatment' (those at the higher end were morbidly obese to start with), but after one year they will have regained some weight and lost only 8–9 per cent, after three years 7 per cent and after four years 5 per cent. The big caveat to this remarkable success (at least for a diet) is that these figures only apply to those who stick with it. Almost half the people in these studies who started a meal-replacement diet had stopped by the six-month stage. These diets work very quickly but are almost impossible to stick to for any length of time, and the weight quickly comes back on (often with interest) once you stop – and apparently even if you don't.

Low-carbohydrate diets

Low-carbohydrate diets take exactly the opposite approach to the other two, insisting on the almost complete elimination of carbohydrates from the diet. The only real difference between the various forms of low-carb diet is the amount of carbohydrate you're permitted. Most of them also insist on 'branding' their diet by requiring you to have certain 'special' foods (that you can usually only obtain with a bag of unmarked small-denomination notes at 'selected health-food stores'). This type of diet is generally sold in bookshops rather than 'wellness centres', supermarkets or pharmacies.

The grandaddy of modern low-carb diets is the Atkins Diet, based on the program set out in *Dr Atkins' Diet Revolution*, a low-carb bible that first appeared in 1972 and has now sold more than 10 million copies worldwide. The simple prescription is to eat as much fat and protein as you wish but severely limit your carbohydrate intake (Dr Atkins suggested a limit of 20 grams per day, which is half a slice of white bread).

Other popular low-carbohydrate diets include:

- *Enter the Zone* by Barry Sears & Bill Lawren (Regan Books, 1995)
- *Protein Power* by Michael R. Eades & Mary Dan Eades (Bantam, 1996)
- *The Paleo Diet* by Loren Cordain (John Wiley & Sons, 2002)
- *The South Beach Diet* by Arthur Agatston (Rodale, 2003)
- *The Thyroid Diet* by Mary J. Shomon (HarperCollins, 2004)
- *The CSIRO Total Wellbeing Diet* by Peter Clifton & Manny Noakes (Penguin, 2005)
- *Bodytrim* by Geoff Jowett (Igea Life Sciences, 2007)
- *The Dukan Diet* by Pierre Dukan (Hodder & Stoughton, 2010; first published in France in 2000).

In a strict sense, low-carb dieters are not calorie-counters. They don't know or care what the calorie content of their food is. But the reality is that by eliminating something that for most people makes up about half of their normal diet (or more, if they're following the 'healthy eating' guidelines), they're severely limiting the number of things they can eat. The diet seeks to eliminate the bottom of the healthy eating pyramid almost completely, which pretty much leaves meat, eggs and milk.

Do low-carb diets actually work?

Studies on the effectiveness of low-carb diets generally reveal that the low-carbers end up eating the same number of calories as low-fat dieters. In general, whether the dieter is substituting carbohydrates for fat or fat for carbohydrates, they're simply reducing their daily calorie intake.

The low-carbers do, however, have one advantage that might explain the popularity of their approach. By eliminating carbohydrates, they also eliminate the swings in blood-sugar concentration associated with carbohydrate consumption. When our blood sugar starts to get too low, a hormone called glucagon is released. This stimulates a hunger signal, ultimately making our upper intestine contract and our tummies gurgle. This is why most people following low-fat – and therefore high-carbohydrate – diets report feeling hungry all the time. But when low-carbers remove carbohydrates from their diet, their body switches to greater reliance on fatty acids and ketones manufactured from protein for its energy, and so one of the primary hunger signals is suppressed. The result is that most people who follow low-carbohydrate diets report not feeling hungry. Both types of diet get to the same place (reduced calorie intake), it's just that the low-carbers probably enjoy the whole experience a little more.

The other advantage of low-carb diets is on the bathroom scales. Our bodies use carbohydrates called glycogen, 'animal starch' or 'brown fat' as a quick-access energy store in our liver and muscles. When we stop eating carbohydrates, our body quickly uses up the glycogen before it starts working on the normal fat stores. Glycogen is a carbohydrate, so it's stored with water. When we lose the brown fat, we also lose the water, so a low-carb diet produces a pretty magical and instantaneous weight-loss result right at the start, which the average dieter finds fairly motivating.

Studies on low-carb versus low-fat diets

In 2003, a group of doctors from four US medical schools decided it was time for some hard evidence on diet effectiveness. They set up a test of the two major diet theories and had a low-carb diet face off against a low-fat (or calorie-restriction) diet. They rounded up 63 obese Americans who were otherwise healthy and divided them randomly into low-carbers and calorie-counters. The study was much more like the real world than the studies described earlier. Nobody was having their meals or weekly counselling sessions bought for them.

The low-carbers were instructed to follow the Atkins Diet for a year and the calorie-counters were told to follow a standard high-carbohydrate, low-fat, low-calorie diet consistent with the traditional food pyramid (60 per cent carbohydrate, 25 per cent fat, 15 per cent protein).

As the graph shows, after six months things were going great for the low-carb group. From an average starting weight of just under 99 kilograms they'd managed to lose an average of 7 kilograms. The low-fat folks had lost about half as much – 3.2 kilograms. Neither group had lost weight at anything like the rate predicted by calorie consumption alone.

Unfortunately, the six-month win was as good as it was going to get. Both groups then started steadily putting weight back on. By the 12-month mark (when the study ended) their average weight loss was a mere 4.4 kilograms for the low-carbers and just 2.5 kilograms for the fat-watchers, which was not even statistically significant, meaning the difference was so small it could have been due to chance alone. Mathematically, they should both have lost 32 kilograms after a year, but neither group managed to keep even 5 per cent of their body weight off. All were obese before undertaking a year of significant deprivation and all were obese afterwards. It was hardly a resounding success for either approach to dieting.

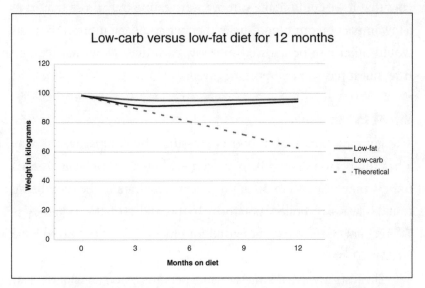

Produced from data presented in Foster *et al.*, 'A Randomised Trial of a Low-Carbohydrate Diet for Obesity', *New England Journal of Medicine*, 2003.

The low-GI diet

The low-carb diet sounds like magic. The only problem is that it's very hard to stick to. We live in a society where there's almost no food without carbohydrates and everyone around us is chowing down on the stuff (even a sausage roll is one-quarter carbs). Because of this, some enterprising folks have come up with the low-carb diet you can have when you're not having a low-carb diet. It's called the low-GI (for low glycemic index) diet.

The glycemic index is a measure of how much a given carbohydrate affects our blood-sugar levels. When we eat a carbohydrate, it's converted to blood glucose over time. This causes a spike and then a decline in the amount of glucose circulating in our bloodstream. The thinking is that not all carbohydrate foods are equal. Some (such as white bread or pure glucose) keep our blood-sugar levels higher for longer than others (such as porridge). The theory goes that if we could make sure we were eating only those that have a low impact on our blood sugar, then we could eat more carbs than would otherwise be allowed in a low-carb diet. Now that may be true, but it has some important caveats.

What is the GI?

The glycemic index of a food is measured by comparing the way a healthy person responds to 50 grams of glucose (or white bread) to how they respond to 50 grams of carbohydrate in the food being tested – let's say boiled potatoes. If the effect of the potatoes is 70 per cent of the effect measured for glucose, then it's said to have a GI of 70.

The tests involve taking the same person's blood constantly over several hours on different days for each food, so it's a very involved process. We know that anything else eaten with the tested food will significantly affect the outcome. If our potatoes are mashed and served with butter, or baked and served with diced bacon, the combination will likely have a lower GI. How much lower? It's anybody's guess, because it would be extraordinarily difficult to measure all the possible combinations (and that's before we even consider the fact that we don't generally eat foods on their own). Steak might come with the potato and honey might come with the bread. No one has any idea whatsoever what the GI of even those combinations might be, let alone the possible mix of everything a person eats in a day.

The other thing we know about GI is that no two people react in the same way to a particular carbohydrate. This is why the test has to be performed on the same person on different days – they'd probably feel like a pincushion by the end of a test for 10 foods! So just because the healthy person who did the test got a GI of 70 for a boiled potato, doesn't mean that the obese chap sitting next to you on the bus would get the same number.

And just in case you're wondering if a low-GI diet does any better in weight-loss studies, a recent shoot-out between a low-GI and a standard low-calorie diet suggests they're both as useless as each other when it comes to losing weight. At the end of that trial, which only ran for 36 weeks, the people in the low-GI camp had lost 2.8 kilograms and the calorie-counters had lost 2.2 kilograms, and both groups regained the weight quickly.

The dangers of GI

GI is an interesting academic exercise but it's not a harmless one. It has a hidden danger in that the carbohydrate it assigns the lowest and therefore the best GI rating is fructose (it has a GI of 19). Fructose does not produce a significant blood-sugar response because it's invisible to the hormone system that controls our appetite. This means that table sugar, which is half fructose, has a much lower GI than you might expect (55–65, where 55 is considered to be a low-GI food). One of the most effective ways to lower the GI rating of a processed food is to add sugar. Fat also lowers the GI. So, for best results, food processors often add fat and sugar. This is how products such as Nutella (half sugar and a third fat, with a GI of 33) come up so well on a GI-ranking table.

The GI-lowering capability of fructose and the fact that it's much sweeter than sugar means that food manufacturers are increasingly using pure fructose rather than sugar to sweeten products. This allows them to make three fabulous health claims all in one go: suddenly the product contains 'no cane sugar' is 'low-GI' and has less sugar per serve.

A GI rating for food might help an insulin-dependent diabetic plan how much insulin they're likely to need to inject after eating a certain type of food (the higher the GI, the more insulin they'll probably need). But its significant blind spot for fructose means that following such a diet is likely to cause them long-term harm (see Chapter 6 for much more detail on this) and make their insulin dependence worse over time. Low-GI diets are often thought of as low-carb for folks who don't really want to go low-carb, but the problems associated with how the ratings are calculated, combined with the danger of the diet encouraging overconsumption of fructose, mean that such diets are not just useless, they're also extremely dangerous.

Calorie-restriction diets really don't work

In 2007 Traci Mann and her colleagues from the University of California, Los Angeles analysed the outcomes of long-term randomised studies of calorie-restriction diets, which include all of the types of diets discussed above. They were able to find only seven sufficiently rigorous long-term studies that ran for two years or more. In those studies, the average weight loss at the end for the people on the diets was just 1.1 kilograms (and trending down), while the controls (those people not on any of the diets) gained 0.6 kilograms over the same period.

Probably the best thing that could be said about all the diets studied was that they slowed the small weight gain that would otherwise have occurred. When dieters were followed for four or five years, their rate of weight gain didn't appear to level off in the way it did for non-dieters, suggesting that a diet puts a dint in a cycle of continuous weight gain but doesn't make any real long-term (greater than two-year) difference. Mann and her colleagues concluded that, statistically speaking, the best indicator that someone will be heavier in five years' time is them being on a diet now.

Fatness is a condition that affects two-thirds of adults and one-third of children. In Australia we spend the better part of a billion of our hard-earned after-tax dollars on solutions to that problem, and yet there's absolutely no evidence that anything we buy actually works.

Doctors can't get away with prescribing drugs that do nothing. Lawyers can't sell legal services that do nothing (most of the time), mechanics can't charge you for fixing your car and not do it. But for some reason, when it comes to the diet industry, we've been so conditioned to believe that failure is our fault, we almost expect to fail. An ingrained part of these diets is their requirement for willpower. If the diet doesn't work, it's not the fault of the diet, but simply that we're weak in the willpower department (almost by definition, we're lacking in willpower if we're fat enough to require a diet in the first place). So if the diet doesn't work, they say, it's because we gave in to our sloth and gluttony and refused to suffer enough.

Is weight-loss surgery an option?

When the diets inevitably fail, modern medicine has one last throw of the dice for the so-called chronically slothful and gluttonous – bariatric surgery. And the most popular bariatric surgery in Australia today by a country mile is lap-band surgery. In 2007, just 8193 lap-band procedures were performed in Australia, but by 2008 this had grown to 12247, a whopping 50 per cent increase in the market in just one year. In 2010, just over 14000 lap-band procedures were performed in Australia, even though very little of the cost is covered by Medicare rebates – the average out-of-pocket cost for the recipients was $13000.

The idea behind lap-band surgery is to restrict the fuel supply without the need for willpower. It's like clamping a fuel line in a car – less fuel gets through for a given squeeze of the accelerator. But our bodies are nothing if not adaptive, so they just push harder and longer on the accelerator, ramping up their demand for calories.

Bariatric surgery is not a simple piece of cosmetic beautification. This is significant surgery that requires major reoperation in 20 per cent of cases. For more than half of recipients, it doesn't result in significant weight loss at all. For most, the surgery has only a 40 per cent chance of triggering a remission of type 2 diabetes (and then only for a maximum of nine years), and patients only gain an extra 1.2 years of life expectancy. And these are the best possible outcomes, because they're the results of trials funded by the manufacturer of the lap-banding devices itself. Independent verification of any of these results is sorely lacking.

Not even the most fanatical supporter of bariatric surgery would suggest that it even remotely attempts to treat the cause of obesity. Bariatric surgery is the socially acceptable version of stitching someone's lips together with wire. It pays no heed to the metabolic dysfunction that caused that person to overeat in the first place, it just treats (temporarily) the overeating. It changes nothing about what they eat, either, it just requires it to be liquefied so that it fits through the now-tiny path to the stomach.

3. EXERCISE WON'T HELP YOU LOSE WEIGHT, EITHER

Exercising willpower is only one side of the remedy for fatness proposed by those in the know. We're also supposed to exercise, well, ourselves. The Federal Government's official *Dietary Guidelines for Australian Adults* document tells us that to prevent weight gain we need to be physically active. It defines 'physically active' as doing 30 minutes of moderate-intensity exercise a day. It doesn't go so far as to promise weight loss from exercise, but it does suggest we won't get fat if we exercise frequently. This has been translated into an 'exercise will make you lose weight (as long as you suffer enough)' message that's shouted from every street corner, mostly by folks who have a buck to make from convincing us to sweat like pigs. The health-equipment, gym and weight-loss industries have all gone from being worth zero to billions of dollars in the last 30 years. Forget the internet boom; the boom in the 'health' industry has been sustained like nothing in our economic history.

According to the Australian Sports Commission, in 2009, more than two-thirds (69.5 per cent) of us exercised at least once a week, almost half (47.7 per cent) participated in sport three or more times a week and almost a third (28 per cent) were hitting the sports field five or more days a week. We should treat these numbers with caution, however, as they're based on self-completed survey forms (and we all tend to exercise more when filling out surveys!). Money may be a more reliable indicator. According to the Australian Bureau of Statistics, in 2004 we spent almost 20 per cent more on physical activity than in 1998, including a whopping 92 per cent increase in the number of gym memberships. Even in the US, where all kinds of unwelcome records are being set for obesity, the National Federation of State High School Associations reports that the number of students participating in high-school athletics has just increased for the 19th consecutive year. And it's not just the kids. Their parents have been spending up big on sports gear, too. Since 2000, US sporting apparel sales have gone up 35.3 per cent and sports shoe sales are up 44.2 per cent, while between 1990 and 2008, sports equipment sales more than doubled, from US$30 billion to almost US$70 billion.

How exercise got tied up with weight loss

Exercise is now so tightly bound with weight loss in the minds of governments, educators and the public that to challenge the suggestion appears as foolhardy as arguing that the sky is not really blue. But this 'truth' is in reality a very recent phenomenon. The common belief that exercise causes weight loss can be traced to one very influential nutritionist, Jean Mayer. A French-born hero of the Resistance, Mayer moved to the US just after World War II. He worked at the UN Food and Agriculture Organization in Washington, DC while earning a doctorate in physiological chemistry at Yale (with a dissertation on the relationship between vitamins A and C in rats). After earning his PhD, he joined Harvard's newly founded Department of Nutrition and became a prolific and high-profile publisher of papers and books on hunger, nutrition and the then-emerging public health problem of obesity.

In 1959 the *New York Times* credited Mayer with destroying the theory that exercise had nothing to do with losing weight. Until that time, doctors had pretty much uniformly believed that exercising just made you hungrier. One leading medical textbook at the time even famously quoted a study showing that lumberjacks ate twice as much as tailors and concluded that 'Vigorous muscle exercise usually results in immediate demand for a large meal'. Many studies had shown that patients lost more weight if they lay in bed than if they pursued vigorous exercise. It was an accepted tenet of medical practice that prescribing exercise to treat obesity was akin to prescribing beer to treat alcoholism. All the prescription did was make the obese person hungrier and therefore more likely to overeat.

Dr Mayer's populist writings during the 1960s changed all this. He published article after article showing that obese people were less physically active and concluding that being more physically active would make you less fat. Mayer's only test of his theory (on humans) involved a survey of the eating and working habits of 213 workers at a market and mill in India in 1953. The study compared the weight and activity levels of mill workers (who spent the whole day shovelling coal) with market stallholders (who were completely sedentary) and clerks (who did nothing but sit all day). Unsurprisingly, the more active mill workers weighed more and ate more than the less active mill workers. Oddly, though, the more sedentary a clerk or stallholder was, the less they weighed and the more they ate.

The study has never been replicated and could really have been used to prove any point the author wanted to make. Maybe exercise makes us eat more. Maybe eating more makes us exercise. Maybe sitting around makes us eat more. Or perhaps eating more makes us sit around more. But none of this confusion made it into Dr Mayer's findings. He boldly concluded that if we don't exercise enough we'll eat more and get fat. He said his work showed definitively that fat people exercise less than thin people, and that they're fat because they exercise less. As health adviser to three US presidents, he then evangelically pushed this theory into the American and then the world consciousness.

Doctors didn't go down without a fight. As late as 1965, they were still writing to the *New York Times* in response to articles published by Mayer, decrying his exercise theories as nonsensical. But Mayer was by then a hugely influential nutritionist and was on a mission to convince the public that the cure to being fat was exercise – and convince them he eventually did. If only being thin were simply a matter of climbing on a treadmill for an extra half-hour a day, even supposing we did have the time. Unfortunately, as the following example shows, the research once again fails to support the policy-makers.

The truth about exercise

In 2010, an extraordinarily detailed study of Mayer's theory was published in the *British Medical Journal*. The researchers followed 202 children from 40 primary schools in England for up to 10 years. Once a year the children were given accelerometers (to measure activity) to wear for a week and subjected to a battery of physical examinations. The study aimed to determine whether fatness leads to inactivity or inactivity leads to fatness. Just like Jean Mayer, they found that a child who was overweight at age seven was likely to exercise less for the following three years. But the researchers also found that if a kid didn't do any exercise, that fact did not allow them to predict whether the child would be overweight. The sloths got just as fat or stayed just as thin as the kids who spent all day on the move.

The researchers concluded: 'Physical inactivity appears to be the *result* of fatness rather than its *cause*. This reverse causality may explain why attempts to tackle childhood obesity by promoting physical activity have been largely unsuccessful.' In other words, we stop exercising because we're fat. We're not fat because we stop exercising.

This evidence from schoolchildren is backed up by the joint guidelines on physical activity for healthy adults published by the American Heart Association and the American College of Sports Medicine in August 2007. After reviewing all of the available evidence, they recommend 30 minutes of moderate-intensity physical activity five days a week to 'promote and maintain health'. Noticeably absent from the guidelines is any suggestion that exercise would definitely lead to weight reduction. The best they could come up with was: 'It is reasonable to assume that persons with relatively high daily energy expenditures would be less likely to gain weight over time, compared with those who have low energy expenditures. *So far, data to support this hypothesis are not particularly compelling . . .*' (my italics).

The problem with exercise is that it just doesn't burn that many calories. And any calories it does chew through are very easily replaced with microscopic changes in diet. We're exceedingly efficient at using our calories. The 150 calories in a glass of apple juice would let us ride a bicycle 8 kilometres, but the same energy (in petrol) would push a car just 250 metres. As Louis Newburgh of the University of Michigan famously calculated in his 1942 paper on the nature of obesity, a man will burn just 3 calories walking up a flight of stairs. 'He will have to climb twenty flights of stairs to rid himself of the energy contained in one slice of bread!' Newburgh said. A quick bit of maths on a calorie-counter tells us that the average adult male will burn about 100 more calories in 30 minutes of moderate-intensity exercise than in sitting around reading this book. That's about the number of calories in one Monte Carlo biscuit.

Exercise fanatics would respond that it's not the one-off go on the treadmill or flight of stairs that will knock the weight off, it's showing dedication and doing it day in, day out. They'd say if exercise doesn't work for us, it's because we're not sufficiently dedicated to the task (in other words, we're not suffering enough).

Does regular exercise cause weight loss?

A major 2011 study conducted by the University of Pittsburgh set out to prove that if overweight people could just be made to exercise consistently, then weight loss would inevitably follow. The researchers recruited 278 overweight adults aged between 18 and 55 who didn't do regular exercise. They randomly divided the volunteers into three groups. They gave the first group a booklet and a monthly newsletter telling them the benefits of exercise and left them to figure it out for themselves. The other two groups were each given a structured program of high-intensity exercise intended to last either 30 minutes a day (for the moderate group) or 60 minutes a day (for the hard-core group). These groups would also attend weekly help and advice sessions with a trainer, to ensure they were sticking to the program, and could also exercise on-site with the trainer any time they wished. None of the groups was given any information or instructions about diet and they weren't encouraged to count calories.

The study ran for 18 months, an unusually long time for this kind of study. After all that time and effort, however, the results were disappointing to say the least. The first group (the folks with the booklet and an encouraging wave) did pretty well. They averaged about 15 minutes a day of exercise. The folks in the moderate group only managed to exercise for 14 minutes a day, despite all the help – which suggests that their meetings with the trainer were a waste of time and money. The hard-core group did quite a bit better, managing to average 31 minutes of exercise a day, but that was still half what they were supposed to be doing.

On the diet front, everyone in the study took the researchers' advice and didn't worry about it. There were no differences between the groups in terms of their average calorie intake. The percentage of body fat (about 30 per cent) for all three groups was pretty much the same at the end as it was at the start. The first group lost an average of 0.5 kilograms, the moderate group knocked off a whole 0.7 kilograms and the heavy hitters in the hard-core group managed a great big 0.8 kilograms. In fact, there was no statistically significant difference between the groups as to how much weight they lost, which means the results are simply a matter of chance. None of the groups managed to lose one whole kilogram in a year and a half of solid exercising. They were overweight before they started and they were still overweight when they finished.

Averages often hide unpleasant details, and this study is no exception. Just 27 per cent of all participants managed to lose more than 3 per cent of their body weight over 18 months. Almost 53 per cent were the same weight at the end as they were at the start. And they were the lucky ones, because 20 per cent of participants actually managed to gain more than 3 per cent of their body weight (an average of 4 kilograms). Why didn't all this exercise produce significant changes in body weight? Well, if you've ever done any high-intensity exercise (people tell me it's hard work), you already know the answer. In fact, if you've ever skipped lunch so you can have a huge dinner because the boss is paying (much more within my area of expertise), you know the reason too. When we exercise or skip a meal we get hungry. It's called working up an appetite. So when these poor souls pounded the pavement for 18 months for up to 31 minutes a day, all they were really doing was making sure they ate a bit more at their next meal.

Apart from being pointless if weight loss is the aim, exercise is a time thief. Thirty minutes of exercise is not just 30 minutes of exercise. There's the time spent shovelling yourself into the costume (usually consisting of unnaturally large quantities of lycra), the time spent getting to the place of exercise (we seem to prefer to do it where people can see us doing it) and the time spent showering and prettifying after the exercise. Most people won't get any change out of an hour and a half for a half-hour of exercise. And it can all be undone with a two-second chomp on a biscuit.

What exercise does and doesn't do

There are lots of good reasons to exercise. The Mayo Clinic says there are seven benefits to exercise, only one of which is weight control. The others are improving your mood, combating heart disease by improving blood circulation, strengthening your heart and lungs, helping you get a better night's sleep, putting the spark back in your sex life (!), and just for fun. You could exercise because it gives you an endorphin rush. You could do it because it gives you 'headspace' – while you exercise, your mind can wander and be free to get away from the pressures of the day. You could do it for 'you' time – no one's going to criticise you for devoting half an hour to solitary exercise a day. You could just do it to feel well.

So, nothing I've said should suggest that there aren't good health reasons for exercise, merely that weight loss shouldn't be the primary motivating factor. The reality is, our bodies are pretty good at adjusting their energy requirements based on the amount of physical activity we actually do. This is perhaps why the American

Heart Association was struggling to find any evidence that exercise results in weight loss.

Exercise burns so few calories that very few people can commit the time or willpower required for it to seriously affect energy balance. But even if they could, using more energy just increases the demand for energy – any gym junkie could tell you that. Lumberjacks eat more than office workers because they exercise more. Telling us we can control this process with willpower is the same as telling us we can control our body temperature or our shoe size with willpower. It's nonsensical. But that hasn't stopped exercise becoming a central pillar of almost every weight-loss message of the last four decades.

4. VITAMINS – DON'T WASTE YOUR MONEY

The number of us taking vitamin and mineral supplements has risen dramatically in the last three decades. Approximately half of all US adults and more than 63 per cent of those over 60 regularly take supplements. And the numbers are very similar in Australia, with around 43 per cent of adults regularly using supplements. In the year 2000, Australians spent $1.67 billion on dietary supplements. This was four times the amount we spent on prescription drugs and triple the amount we spent just seven years earlier. As our health problems get worse and worse, we increasingly turn to over-the-counter supplements as part of the solution. We want a pill we can pop that makes us think we feel less lethargic or less stressed, or .that makes our children smarter or our bones less brittle. And the supplements industry is only too happy to assure us they have the answer to all that and much more.

Our bodies use 13 vitamins. Twelve are found largely in meat and one is found largely in fruit and vegetables, so anyone telling you to eat fruit and veg for the vitamins has well and truly got the wrong end of the stick. Four of the vitamins (A, D, E, and K) are fat-soluble and nine (the eight B vitamins and vitamin C) are water-soluble. Water-soluble vitamins (see the table below) dissolve in water, are distributed throughout our largely water-based body and are generally excreted in our urine if we consume too much of them. This doesn't mean that overconsumption is harmless, however. Consistently high levels can result in some nasty disease outcomes. We hang onto fat-soluble vitamins (see the table over the page) and very rarely need to top them up from our diet, but once again, over-consumption can have some downright dangerous consequences.

The water-soluble vitamins: things need to get pretty extreme before we're deficient in any of them.

Vitamin	Also known as	Best dietary sources	Deficiency can lead to
B1	thiamine (meaning 'sulfur-containing vitamine')	brown rice, oats, pork; in Australia all flours and cereal products are fortified with thiamine	beriberi (see page 53)
B2	riboflavin (from 'ribose' – the sugar it's based on – and 'flavin' from the Latin *flavus* meaning 'yellow'; this makes our urine turn yellow when we take vitamin B tablets)	liver, chicken, milk, yoghurt, eggs	ariboflavinosis (similar to pellagra, below)
B3	niacin (**ni**cotinic **ac**id vitam**in** – it's derived from nicotine)	liver, chicken, fish, beef, eggs, milk	pellagra (see page 55)

B5	pantothenic acid	liver, chicken, fish, mushrooms, milk, beef	—
B6	pyridoxine	fish, liver, potatoes, nuts, chicken, bananas	—
B7	biotin	everything; and our gut bacteria make more than we need anyway	—
B9	folic acid	chicken, lentils, chick peas, spinach; in Australia all flours and cereal products are fortified with folic acid	deficiency in pregnant women can lead to neural tube birth defects (spina bifida – see page 77)
B12	cobalamin	molluscs, liver, chicken, crabs, fish, beef	decreased cognitive function
C	ascorbic acid	peppers, broccoli, berries, cabbage, fruit	scurvy (see page 58)

The fat-soluble vitamins. To the extent we need to absorb any of these from our food, it's better if we consume the food with fat (butter on your greens, anyone?).

Vitamin	Best dietary sources	Deficiency can lead to
A	meat or, if none is available, carrot, broccoli, sweet potato, butter, spinach, pumpkin	night blindness and impaired immune system (too much during pregnancy can cause birth defects)

D	we make it ourselves when exposed to sunlight, but it's also present in liver, eggs and fish; no plant sources except UV-irradiated mushrooms and yeast; in Australia, margarine must be fortified with vitamin D	rickets
E	we make it ourselves, but it's also present in seed oils	extremely rare and not caused by diet
K	leafy green vegetables (spinach, cabbage, broccoli)	extremely rare and not caused by diet

As the following rundown of the history of vitamin discovery will show, although we need vitamins, that doesn't mean we need to take supplements. One thing you'll notice in the history of vitamin discovery (and of pharmaceutical research in general) is that the answer is always to find a substance that can be sold to the punters, rather than to fix what caused the problem in the first place.

The discovery of vitamins: vitamin B1

The very first vitamin discovered was the one we now call B1 or thiamine. It became necessary to discover it because Europeans started messing with a traditional Asian food source. Beriberi is a wasting disease that starts with lethargy and fatigue and ends in death. For centuries, the problem had been known in Asia as a relatively rare disease that happened when people were starving, but by the late 19th century it had become one of the most common diseases in South-East Asia. In some towns, as many as half the babies died from it. The Dutch colonies that we now call Indonesia were particularly badly hit, and the Dutch administrators were looking hard for a cure. Christiaan Eijkman, a Dutch doctor, joined a mission sent out by the Dutch Government to find one. By 1897,

Eijkman had shown that feeding lab chickens polished (white) rice gave them beriberi but feeding them unpolished rice (with the bran still attached) didn't. He was also able to cure the chickens he'd made sick just by giving them brown rice.

The reason beriberi had so suddenly become a problem was that the Dutch had been innovative with the food supply. When steam-driven mills first became available in the late 19th century, the Dutch applied them to the polishing of rice in their colonies. Until then, the traditional method of rice preparation was to remove the hard outer husk using a hulling machine, which was essentially a drum that banged all the rice together. The hulled rice was very much like our brown rice of today – the outer protective layer is removed but the smear of brown bran is still intact. The new mills could polish away the bran – and the associated nutty taste – and produce perfect white rice. The only problem was that the bran layer clearly contained something that prevented beriberi. And if your only food source was that rice, as it was for most of the indigenous population, eliminating the 'something' meant the development of deficiencies and ultimately beriberi.

In 1906, Sir Frederick Hopkins, a British biochemist, followed up on Eijkman's work and theorised that there was more to food than mere carbohydrates, protein and fat. He thought that some sort of 'accessory factor' in the rice bran was necessary to avoid beriberi (he later shared the Nobel Prize in Medicine with Eijkman for that little guess). The race was then on to isolate the anti-beriberi factor so it could be sold as a treatment. A supplement that would have to be sold to all inhabitants of South-East Asia was a prize worth finding.

In 1912, Kazimierz Funk, a Polish biochemist, thought he'd discovered the mystery substance when he isolated an amine (a chemical compound of nitrogen) from the rice bran. Funk called his discovery *vitamine* ('vital' + 'amine'). It wasn't until 1926 that the correct chemical, vitamin B1 or thiamine, was isolated in pure form.

Around this time it became clear both that there were other 'vitamines' and that they need not be amines, so vitamines became vitamins. By 1936, scientists were able to manufacture artificial vitamin B1 and the supplements industry was born. After World War II, most white rice was supplemented with vitamin B1 and the beriberi problem disappeared almost immediately. In Australia (but not New Zealand), baking flour is now enriched with vitamin B1, even though there's never been a beriberi problem in this country.

The discovery of vitamin B3

Beriberi wasn't the only disease caused by vitamin deficiencies. At around the time the Dutch were sorting out their little problem in the colonies, a very nasty disease was reaching epidemic proportions in the United States. Pellagra (from the Italian *pelle* – 'skin' and *agra* – 'sour') is beriberi for people whose diet is based on corn rather than rice. The symptoms of this horrible disease are described as the four Ds: diarrhoea, dermatitis, dementia and ultimately death – untreated, a sufferer will die within five years.

The disease was an intermittent problem in the 17th and 18th centuries in southern Europe, where the inhabitants were dependent upon corn for survival. When cheap American corn was introduced and replaced traditional wheat or rye, food yield per acre increased dramatically, and more food meant more people could be fed from the same amount of land. The population of Spain, southern France, northern Italy, Romania and southern Russia exploded, and wherever corn went, pellagra followed. Because pellagra only occurred in areas where corn was the staple crop, it was thought to be caused by corn spoilage. But strangely, in the Americas, indigenous people had lived on corn for thousands of years without any pellagra at all.

When pellagra cases appeared in the immigrant American population in 1902, doctors were mystified as to the causes. By 1907, cases were occurring with alarming frequency in prisons and orphanages. In the 1907–11 period, almost 16000 cases and 6205 deaths were reported in the southern states of the US. In mental hospitals, pellagra was now causing more deaths than tuberculosis. By 1915, 75000 new cases a year were being reported, and during the 1920s this annual rate rose to 100000, with the nine southern states accounting for more than 90 per cent of cases. It was a full-blown epidemic, the likes of which most Americans had never seen. In the period 1906–30, pellagra was reported in 3 million people and caused more than 100000 deaths. For comparison, Australia lost approximately the same number of troops during World Wars I and II combined.

In 1914, the US Surgeon General assigned Dr Joseph Goldberger to study the disease. Goldberger had been with the US National Health Service for most of his 15-year career, screening immigrants for yellow fever, dengue fever and typhoid fever. Goldberger knew a lot about infectious diseases caused by microbes, and he was pretty sure that, despite the prevailing medical wisdom, pellagra was nothing of the sort. He quickly guessed that it was linked to poverty and a poor diet, an observation that didn't go down well in the southern states. One of his key observations was that in mental hospitals, only the patients, never the staff, had pellagra, from which he surmised it could not be infectious. That the staff ate at the same institution seemed to be a setback to his theory that pellagra was diet-related, until he noticed a very important detail – the staff always ate first.

The monotonous institutional diet consisted of meat (largely pork), cornmeal mush (a sort of porridge made from corn) and molasses. This meal was known at the time as the 3M diet – meat, meal and molasses. Because the staff had first choice, they took most of the meat, leaving the inmates with a diet very similar to that of most of the poorest inhabitants of the south – cornmeal and molasses (I guess that would be the 2M diet). In orphanages, he noticed that children given milk were fine but those who lived on the 2M diet without milk got pellagra. He quickly obtained funding for a trial of introducing milk at two orphanages and the pellagra cleared up immediately. Goldberger knew he was onto something: pellagra was certainly a disease of the diet and not an infection.

At that time, microbial causes for some of the most lethal diseases (typhoid, tuberculosis, meningitis, cholera, malaria, scarlet fever and tetanus, to name a few) were being discovered at the rate of about one a year. The medical profession 'knew' pellagra was the same, and they lampooned Goldberger as a nutcase. The vilification drove him to some pretty extreme experiments: he had himself and his wife injected with the blood of sufferers (called pellagrins); and he and his lab workers ate bread dough impregnated with faeces and dried urine from pellagrins. This made them all very sick, but not from pellagra. His strange antics eventually got him what he wanted: he convinced the authorities to allow him to feed a group of prisoners a 2M diet and induce pellagra. His prison experiment was a success and the cause and the cure were clear. The only problem now was money.

Goldberger knew the cure to pellagra lay in a better diet, but the political response was that the economy of the south couldn't afford to improve the diet of inmates, let alone the population as a whole, so he set about trying to find the single factor, which he called PPF for 'pellagra preventing factor', so that it could be given as a supplement. Almost by accident, he happened upon the magical curative powers of brewer's yeast. In dogs, pellagra manifests as something called 'black tongue', which stops the dog swallowing.

Farmers had known for decades that the cure for black tongue was to give the dog some brewer's yeast (it was first tried because yeast was known to stimulate a sick dog's appetite). Goldberger tried giving yeast to pellagra patients and the cure was instantaneous. At last he had found a cheap and easily distributed substance that would prevent pellagra. By the 1940s, the disease had been virtually eliminated in the US.

Goldberger died in 1929 before his PPF – what we now call vitamin B3 or niacin – was isolated, but he'd put the researchers on the right track. Just as with beriberi, the problem was narrowed down to a vitamin deficiency. The difference was that this time it was caused by Europeans deleting something from food preparation rather than adding a new process (such as steam-milling rice).

For millennia, the indigenous peoples of North and South America had treated corn with lime before eating it. Europeans could see no apparent benefit in the lime treatment, and so they deleted it from the process. But the science ultimately proved that lime treatment makes vitamin B3 available to humans, although the fact that indigenous Americans ate a lot more than corn probably had a lot more to do with the absence of pellagra than did the lime treatment. Once again, the Western 'cure' was to discover a supplement and sell it to the sufferers rather than fix the process that caused the problem in the first place.

The discovery of vitamin C

The next vitamin to be discovered wasn't found because of a plague. It wasn't that hundreds of thousands of people were dying from scurvy, but those who did die were pretty important to business. On a ship that has a job to do, losing 20 people is just as inconvenient as losing half the population of an Indonesian island or a southern US town.

Humans have known from the beginnings of recorded history (and probably well before) that if our diet lacks fresh plant food or fresh meat, in three to six months we develop scurvy. This pretty horrible disease begins with brown spots appearing on the skin and then there's bleeding from the gums and all mucous membranes (the nostrils, mouth, lips, eyelids, ears, anus and genitals). It usually ends in death, so it's definitely something to avoid. The symptoms of scurvy are all associated with the manufacture of poor-quality collagen. The mucous membranes are no longer up to the job of holding the body together, the capillaries become too fragile and then bleeding occurs in multiple sites.

It takes a pretty rare combination of circumstances for a human to have no access to fresh food for long enough for it to matter. They have to avoid it completely for more than two months, because even the smallest dose is enough to prevent scurvy. The only time in recent history that humans have managed to induce scurvy is when the British Navy locked up sailors in sailing ships for months on end on a diet of dried biscuits and rum. By the time Captain Cook got under way to 'discover' Australia, they'd figured out that adding cabbage or lime juice (hence the term 'limeys') to the mix sorted out the scurvy problem.

By the early 1930s it was well established that the cure for scurvy was vitamin C or ascorbic acid, and that the best place to get it was fresh food. This means anything other than grains, which are just about the only food completely deficient in vitamin C.

Studies conducted on British conscientious objectors during World War II showed that just 10 milligrams of vitamin C per day are necessary to prevent scurvy symptoms (the amount found in one very small broccoli floret, one small strawberry, a third of a potato or three slices of pizza). Subsequent studies have shown that the threshold is around 7–8 milligrams per day. We'd really have to work hard not to receive an adequate dose of vitamin C just from eating normally, even if our diet consisted of nothing but pizza and chips.

Is there any point taking vitamin C supplements?

Vitamin C is probably the celebrity of vitamins. Most Australian children know of it because most of them, at some stage in their life, have enjoyed chomping on the orange lolly handed out with breakfast. Most plants and animals (except primates and guinea pigs) can make vitamin C from glucose. According to folks studying our genetic code, we lost the ability to make vitamin C around 60 million years ago, at around the same time we lost the ability to break down uric acid. I was busy that day, so I'm not sure why it happened, but one theory is that because ascorbic acid (vitamin C) and uric acid are both powerful anti-oxidants and perform very similar functions in humans, we just took a bit of a shortcut. Our ancestors were making plenty of uric acid (as a by-product of consuming the fructose in fruit and vegetables) and getting plenty of vitamin C from the fruit and veg in their diet, so why would they bother making vitamin C?

Besides being an anti-oxidant, the main role of vitamin C is to assist in the formation of collagen. Collagen, a fibrous, elongated protein, is what our skin, muscles and connective tissues are made of. Since we're 25–35 per cent collagen, we're constantly making and repairing the stuff. We can still make collagen without vitamin C, but it's a second-rate, unstable product. And this is why the symptoms of scurvy all relate to the breakdown of collagen.

Vitamin C is present in just about every food except pasteurised milk (because the heat destroys the vitamin) and we keep a pretty big on-board reservoir handy. An adult male stores about 1800 milligrams of vitamin C and would use 10–30 milligrams a day, which is why it takes two months for scurvy to appear. Our diet needs to be extraordinarily lacking for us to become deficient in vitamin C. The average vitamin C tablet contains 500 milligrams of vitamin C, about a month's worth for an adult male. Just like the rest of the water-soluble vitamins, any excess vitamin C we consume swiftly ends up in our urine.

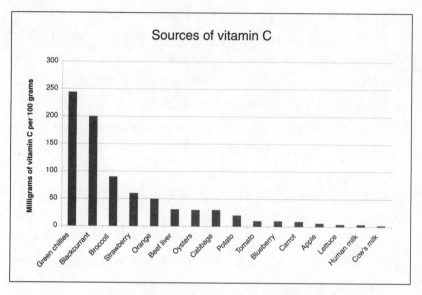

Vitamin C is in just about everything, but it's fragile. These numbers are for raw foods. If the food is cooked the amount is reduced by 60 per cent.

Discovering vitamin A

Beriberi, pellagra and scurvy were big wins for the vitamin-as-a-cure camp. Vitamin research started to ramp up. Who knew what else might be cured by extracting a critical vitamin? There was money to be made in the hunt for vitamin cures.

In 1916, two American research teams racing each other in the vitamin gold rush discovered independently that cow's milk contains something they called 'fat-soluble factor A'. In a follow-up to the beriberi studies, they discovered that rats fed skim milk rather than full-fat milk developed an eye disease called xeroph-thalmia. They found that rats given butter got better immediately and decided there must be a fat-soluble vitamin in milk and butter. It turns out that vitamin A or retinol plays an important role in embryo development, particularly in the growth of the spinal cord and backbone, limbs, heart, eye and ears. The other major function of vitamin A is to switch on the genes that make immature skin cells grow into mature skin cells. By doing this it keeps our skin healthy (which is one reason it's often advertised as a feature of face and hand creams). But it's probably most famous for providing us with the ability to see in low light and in colour.

Vitamin A is critical to our survival, so we're very good at getting all we need from our food supply. It's only found in foods of animal origin, but we can use plant chemicals called carotenes to create vitamin A ourselves if no meat is available. One of these carotenes is what makes carrots orange, which is why your mum told you to eat your carrots so you'd see better at night. Because vitamin A is fat-soluble, eating it without fat dramatically reduces our ability to absorb it. This means that vegans and vegetarians are at significantly higher risk of suffering from vitamin A deficiency than those who eat meat.

Discovering vitamin D

The discovery of vitamin A sent researchers scurrying on the hunt for more fat-soluble vitamins. The steroid that was ultimately labelled vitamin D was first identified in 1919 by Sir Edward Mellanby. He was working as a lecturer in medicine at King's College for Women in London when the Medical Research Committee at the college asked him to investigate the cause of rickets, a disease characterised by bone deformity and weakness. Rickets affected primarily poor, dark-skinned children living in the cities of northern England and the northern United States. Mellanby knew of the work on vitamin A and decided to conduct studies on puppies to see if there was another vitamin in fat that might be implicated in rickets.

Mellanby managed to produce rickets in the pups by feeding them the vitamin A experimental diet of skim milk and bread. He added yeast and orange juice to the diet to see if vitamins B or C were the cause, but they had no effect. When he tried the vitamin A cure of butter or cod-liver oil (a popular cure for rickets since the middle of the 19th century) it completely prevented rickets. It's lucky he kept the dogs inside his lab, because if they'd been outside in the sunshine, nothing he fed them or didn't feed them would have induced rickets.

At first they thought that vitamin A was also the cure for rickets, but a further series of experiments by US researchers in 1922 showed that there were two substances in butter and cod-liver oil, only one of which prevented rickets. A year later, three different laboratories simultaneously discovered that rickets could be prevented simply by exposing the animals to sunlight. It turns out we can make the stuff all by ourselves – all we need is a bit of sunshine.

It took until 1936 to isolate vitamin D, and researchers eventually discovered that it was produced by exposing cholesterol stored in the skin to ultraviolet light (and that it's present in trace amounts in animal products because most animals do the same trick). We use something called 7-dehydrocholesterol to make both cholesterol and vitamin D. When 7-dehydrocholesterol in our skin is exposed to the UVB part of sunlight (which is blocked by sunscreens), one of its bonds is broken and it ultimately turns into vitamin D.

Why we need sun

We store only so much 7-dehydrocholesterol per square centimetre of skin and we store less of it the older we get. When it gets turned into vitamin D it's gone until we make some more, so producing vitamin D is all about exposing as much skin as possible to the sun, without sunscreen, and not necessarily exposing it for a long time (put your clothes back on, Granny – arms and legs will be fine).

Things that affect our ability to make vitamin D

Factor	Reduction in vitamin D production
using sunscreen	99 per cent (SPF 15+)
skin colour	up to 99 per cent
age	up to 75 per cent in a 70-year-old
latitude and season	up to 100 per cent in winter above or below 35 degrees latitude (north of Atlanta in the US, anywhere in Europe or south of Melbourne in Australia)
glass	100 per cent – UVB does not penetrate glass, so we need to get outdoors

Unfortunately, the massive increase in melanoma during the last century has been blamed on sunshine (with very little foundation; see Chapter 10). The result has been public health campaigns using overly simplistic messages about staying out of the sun and ensuring we're slathered in sun cream if we should dare to venture forth.

We've been listening and we've never been so diligent at avoiding the sun. Children aren't allowed to play outside at school without a hat and sunscreen. Most people at the beach now wear bathing suits that cover almost everything, and hats and long-sleeved shirts are de rigueur for all outdoor activities. The problem is that this kind of behaviour also ensures we don't produce sufficient vitamin D.

There's no doubt that prolonged sun exposure will result in skin cancer. But efficient vitamin D production requires regular exposure of large areas of skin for short periods of time. So the health message needs to be more sophisticated than simply saying 'stay out of the sun'. We should regularly get short periods of sun on as much skin as we can (decently) expose.

The darker your skin, the older you are or the further you are from the equator, the longer you'll need to be in the sun to manufacture the same amount of vitamin D. If you're young, white, live north of Melbourne, and expose your arms and legs (without sunscreen) to sunlight in the middle of the day for five minutes twice a week, your body will make all the vitamin D it needs. If you're in your 60s or 70s, living in Melbourne or Tasmania and have darker skin, then you'll need 30 minutes twice a week.

Several large trials in the last decade have detected a very strong inverse association between vitamin D levels, heart disease and various cancers. In other words, the less vitamin D a person has, the higher their risk of developing heart disease and/or cancer. A series of large studies has observed that people who don't go out in the sun much or who wear sun block (and therefore don't make much vitamin D) might have a lower than expected blood-cholesterol level. Low blood cholesterol inevitably leads to increased risks of heart disease and cancer (see Chapter 9), especially if it's combined with a diet that's high in polyunsaturated fats or sugar (or both, just for good measure).

During the 1930s, children living in the cold, dark reaches of England and the United States were routinely given cod-liver oil to prevent rickets. But there's no need to start lining the kids up for their daily dose today. Once vitamin D was isolated, most countries decided to fortify milk with it and the disease was virtually eliminated. To this day, Australian milk is fortified with vitamin D.

Vitamin D is vital for efficient calcium uptake and rickets is caused by lack of calcium, which makes the bones brittle and deformed. Without vitamin D, we can drink milk till the cows come home and very little of the calcium will make its way into our skeleton. Only living things with skeletons bother making vitamin D, so the only dietary sources (besides making it ourselves) are animal-based. Vitamin D also regulates more than 200 genes, and immune cells and brain, prostate, breast and colon tissues all have receptors for it, although we're not sure why. We do know that vitamin D suppresses cell reproduction in normal and cancerous cells. So it does an awful lot and we understand very few of its functions and interactions, but that hasn't stopped us adding it to our food supply en masse as a cure for the consequences of telling everyone to stay out of the sun. As so often in the past, our first solution is to invent a supplement to sell rather than prevent the problem occuring in the first place.

The discovery of folate

The next vitamin to be discovered wasn't part of the vitamin gold rush. It was found because a woman cared enough about other women to doggedly figure out a vitamin-based cure to a deadly deficiency. Dr Lucy Wills attended one of the first English boarding schools prepared to teach boys-only subjects (such as mathematics) to girls. At Cheltenham College for Young Ladies, she was taught by Dorothea Beale, one of the earliest champions for women's voting rights and the founder of the first women's college at Oxford, St Hilda's.

Wills went on to Newnham College at Cambridge, where she received a double-first honours degree in botany and geology in 1911. A stint working as a volunteer hospital nurse in South Africa during World War I pushed her to decide on a career in medicine, which had only very recently become an option for women in England. She returned to London and entered the London School of Medicine for Women.

She graduated in 1920 and took a job in the Department of Chemical Pathology at the Royal Free Hospital. She worked there as part of a team studying the metabolism of pregnant women. She was soon in regular touch with the leading lights of the feminist movement (as it then was in all but name) and in particular with Dr Margaret Balfour, another medical pioneer, in the Indian colonies. Balfour was trying to get to the bottom of why anaemia of pregnancy was so common among Indian textile workers. Anaemia is a class of diseases characterised by a lack of red blood cells, and in pregnancy in particular it can be fatal. The disease was causing extraordinary suffering in the maternity wards of India at the time, and Balfour needed the help of an expert in the metabolism of pregnant women to try to figure out the cause. By the late 1920s, Wills had begun a series of trips to India to help Balfour.

Her comprehensive surveys found that only the poorest manual workers became sick with anaemia during pregnancy. Even then, it only occurred among women who were Hindu – and therefore vegetarian – and whose diet was limited to only a small number of vegetables that provided nowhere near enough calories for a pregnant mother. She at first thought the cause might be a vitamin A or C deficiency, but when she analysed her dietary survey data closely, she found no association between fruit and vegetable consumption and anaemia. She conducted several trials and eventually pinned down the lack of meat as the culprit.

By 1931 she'd figured out that the missing 'Wills factor' (she didn't call it that, it was named in her honour) was the cause, and that the most effective way to ensure the women had sufficient was to feed them liver. She also tried the brewer's yeast that Goldberger had found so effective against pellagra just a decade earlier, only to find it was just as good as the liver and a lot cheaper. Being British, Wills had a compact, cheap and easy-to-administer form of brewer's yeast sitting on her breakfast table every morning – Marmite. She tried it out too and to her delight it worked. She found that anaemic women given Marmite recovered immediately. She didn't know what the Wills factor was or how it worked, but she did know it was present in both liver and the yeast used to make Marmite.

Marmite

Marmite was invented in 1902 as a vegetarian version of Bovril (originally called Johnstone's Fluid Beef – I wonder why they changed that name), a beef extract that was very popular at the time. A yeast extract, it was made from the waste products of the brewery right next door to the factory.

The Marmite Lucy Wills used was British Marmite, which contains half the recommended daily dose of folic acid in about one piece of toast's worth (4 grams) and no sugar. In Australia, the Marmite on sale is New Zealand Marmite, which has 20 per cent less folic acid and is almost 12 per cent sugar.

The Australian version of Marmite is of course Vegemite. It has the same amount of folic acid as New Zealand Marmite but much less (just over 2 per cent) sugar.

By 1945, the Wills factor – now known as folic acid or vitamin B9 – had been isolated in pure form. Folic acid (or folate in its natural state) is critical for the production and repair of DNA molecules and red and white blood cells. Rapidly dividing cells are most vulnerable to folate deficiency, and when the folate supply to bone marrow cells is inadequate, the division of red blood cells becomes abnormal, resulting in fewer but larger red blood cells. This is the type of anaemia Lucy Wills saw in her folate-deficient pregnant mums. Because folate enables rapid cell division and growth (both particularly handy when assembling a baby), a pregnant mother's folate stores are very quickly depleted by the baby's growth. Had those women not been pregnant, they wouldn't have suffered significant problems, even though their diets were extremely low in folate. (For more on the importance of folate in pregnancy, see page 77.)

Vitamins E and K

A few more vitamins were to be discovered, but as with any gold rush, the big nuggets had all been found by the time Lucy Wills started putting Marmite on her patients' toast.

In addition to the water-soluble vitamins B and C, and the fat-soluble vitamins A and D, there are two other fat-soluble vitamins, vitamins E and K. Vitamin E is the name given to a group of powerful anti-oxidants made by our liver (see Chapter 10 for more on the importance of our little vitamin E factory). Some members of this group, called tocopherols, also occur in abundance in seed oils such as sunflower oil, which is why margarines made from these oils are often advertised as having anti-oxidant properties. But as we shall soon see, studies consistently show that supplementing our diet with these anti-oxidants is totally ineffective and may even be harmful.

Vitamin K enables blood coagulation. Pretty much all our needs are supplied by the bacteria inhabiting our colon, and the little we do need is constantly recycled by our body, so we never really use it up and are almost never deficient. Newborn babies are often given a vitamin K shot to tide them over for the first week, while their gut bacteria get up to speed. We get more than enough from any green leafy vegetable (spinach, cabbage, lettuce, broccoli) we accidentally consume (and with my kids, it's likely to be accidental), and we're three times more likely to absorb it from those sources if we also eat fat at the same time.

Can we be vitamin-deficient?

We make all the vitamin E and K we need and can make all the vitamin D we need if we get enough sun. Vitamin A is the only fat-soluble vitamin that really depends on our diet for adequate supplies, but as long as we eat meat, we're extremely unlikely to be deficient. It's theoretically possible to become deficient in some of the water-soluble vitamins (B-group and C), but they were each discovered because a very particular population of people became very ill as a result of very odd diets indeed. If you're planning to become pregnant, then the research suggests that a folic acid supplement is a good idea, not so much to avoid anaemia, which is extremely unlikely with a normal Western diet, but to prevent neural tube defects and spina bifida (see page 77).

If you're a strict vegan, then you're at some risk of vitamin A deficiency if you don't eat enough orange vegetables. And if you're a vegan who stays out of the sun, then vitamin D deficiency is a risk as well. But if, like the vast majority of Australians, you eat a diet that contains meat and even a smattering of fruit or vegetables and occasionally get out in the sun without sunscreen, you're about as likely to need supplements as I am to become Queen of England.

Do vitamins cure cancer?

We're not sold vitamins on the basis that they'll prevent us getting scurvy, beriberi or pellagra. Supplement-sellers know that we know no one suffers from those diseases in Australia today. Vitamins are sold on the basis that they improve our health by curing chronic disease and generally – and very non-specifically – making us feel better or more energetic.

One of the most persistent suggested benefits of vitamins is that they cure cancer or at least help do so. The idea started in 1981 with animal studies that suggested beta-carotene (the vitamin A precursor found in fruits and vegetables) might reduce the risk of cancer.

Two large human trials kicked off in 1985. In Finland, 29 133 male cigarette-smokers were randomly assigned to groups dosed with beta-carotene, vitamin E, both or placebos. The results, reported in 1995, were disastrous. Not only did the beta-carotene groups not enjoy any benefit, but their rates of lung, prostate and stomach cancer were significantly higher.

A similar study kicked off at the same time in the US. The trial involved 18 314 smokers and former smokers. Once again they were assigned to groups taking beta-carotene or vitamin A supplements and groups taking a placebo. The results, reported in 1996, were similar. The folks on the supplements had a 28 per cent greater risk of getting lung cancer and a 46 per cent greater risk of death from lung cancer. Not surprisingly, the suggestion that vitamin A might help with cancer quietly disappeared from the marketing claims.

B-group vitamins also got a guernsey as a cancer treatment in the early 1980s, again based on some very limited animal studies. In 1985, a very large human trial was started in central China, which was chosen because, at the time, vitamin deficiencies (particularly of B-group vitamins) were common, and rates of stomach and throat cancers were exceptionally high. Almost 30 000 people were recruited and assigned to groups supplemented with B-group vitamins (B2 and B3) and placebos. In 1993 the researchers reported a big fat zero. Vitamin B supplements had no effect on cancer rates or cancer deaths, but I guess they could at least be pleased they didn't cause more cancer.

By the early 1990s, research showing that folates (vitamin B9) reduced neural tube defects (see page 77) had been published. Some population studies suggested that people who ate diets including naturally folate-rich foods (such as spinach and chicken) often had lower rates of bowel cancer. A study started in 1994 on 1021 people who'd been diagnosed with benign bowel polyps but didn't have cancer. Polyps are what doctors are looking for when they go 'down there' with a colonoscopy. Polyps are usually benign, but can develop into bowel cancer, so these folks were seen as a good population to test the theory. They took folic acid pills or a placebo for 10 years. The result? Folic acid *increased* the risk of bowel cancer. The study has since been criticised as too small to be definitive, but small or not, the numbers were certainly going in the wrong direction. Claims that vitamin B cures cancer swiftly went the way of the vitamin A claims and slid off the marketing agenda.

In 1993 a couple of studies suggested that vitamin E supplements might lower the risk of heart disease. In the vitamin-marketers' mind it's a small jump from reducing heart disease to curing cancer, so they promoted the claim that vitamin E cures cancer. A 2000 study of almost 10 000 people revealed that vitamin E had no effect on heart disease, while a meta-study of the 19 vitamin E trials conducted before 2005 and involving more than 135 000 people revealed that, in fact, overall death rates were higher in groups taking vitamin E supplements for the treatment of cancer.

The scientific consensus is that vitamin E is just as useless as vitamins A, B and C (see below) for curing cancer, and some of them may indeed be harmful. So since about 2005, vitamin D has been touted as the next big cure, although the evidence bucket is once again looking very empty indeed. A review published in 2011 of more than 1000 studies of vitamin D and calcium supplementation concluded there's no persuasive evidence that vitamin D affects our chances of contracting or dying from cancer. The story was the same for studies focusing on links between vitamin D and heart disease, diabetes and autoimmune diseases – there's no convincing evidence that taking vitamin D in a supplement makes the slightest bit of difference.

I'm waiting with bated breath for the announcement, surely due any time now, that vitamin K cures cancer. The science so far suggests that when we first hear that, we should treat it with just a bit of scepticism.

Is vitamin C a miracle cure?

In the 1980s, theories about vitamin C and cancer were also circulating, driven almost singlehandedly by Linus Pauling, an eminent theoretical physicist and chemist who won the 1954 Nobel Prize in Chemistry for his work on the electrical properties of atomic bonds. He also picked up the 1962 Nobel Peace Prize for proving that above-ground nuclear testing was causing significant rises in radioactive particles in babies' teeth across the United States. His work resulted in the cessation of above-ground testing and the 1963 signing of a partial test-ban treaty between the United States and the Soviet Union.

Pauling was clearly no dummy, so when he became obsessed with what he called megavitamin therapy, people listened. He believed that enormous daily doses of vitamins were the key to good health. In 1970, he published his first popular book, *Vitamin C and the Common Cold*, which recommended daily doses of vitamin C to ward off common colds and generally extend life (yes, that's where that persistent little marketing message comes from). A comprehensive 2007 review of the evidence from placebo-controlled trials concluded that, for most of us, taking vitamin C supplements regularly has absolutely no effect on our chances of catching a cold or the flu. The only exception was that people exposed to extreme physical stress (marathon runners, soldiers on exercises in the Arctic and cross-country skiers in the Swiss Alps) can halve their chances of getting the sniffles if they take a regular dose of vitamin C.

While taking vitamin C regularly doesn't stop ordinary people getting a cold, it does on average reduce the duration of the cold by 8 per cent for adults (meaning the cold would last for 12 days rather than 13) and 13 per cent for children (11.5 days rather than 13), but this only happens if the vitamin is taken *before* the infection starts. Taking vitamin C after you already have a cold makes absolutely no difference to the duration of the symptoms.

In 1979, Pauling published his theory that vitamin C also cured cancer, as a result of which vitamin C was included in the Chinese trial of vitamin B (see above). The result was exactly the same – nothing. Vitamin C supplementation did not affect cancer outcomes or death rates. The result was definitive, but it never quite killed off the marketing message that vitamin C might be a good insurance policy against cancer.

Do vitamins cure heart disease (or anything else)?

Many of us treat vitamins like an insurance policy. We see the marketing about them being full of anti-oxidants, giving us more energy and generally making us healthier, so we figure it can't hurt to self-medicate with the occasional vitamin supplement.

The B-group vitamins and heart disease

One of the major supposed health benefits for the B-group vitamins is that they lower the risk of heart disease. A deficiency in many of the B-group vitamins (but particularly B6, B9 and B12) will result in higher levels of the blood protein homocysteine.

Numerous studies have shown that people with persistently high levels of homocysteine are more likely to have heart disease. We manufacture homocysteine ourselves, but the presence or absence of B-group vitamins seems to affect how much we make. This is where marketers get the claim that B-group vitamins help reduce heart disease, but the association between homocysteine and heart disease is really just an observation, and so far no credible reason for this has come to light.

Several major trials have aimed to reduce heart-disease and stroke outcomes with B-group supplements, but so far there's no evidence that they make the slightest difference. One of the most recent studies is the ongoing VITATOPS trial being conducted by investigators from Royal Perth Hospital in Australia. In 2010, they reported that after two years of B-vitamin supplementation, homocysteine levels were dramatically reduced. Unfortunately, the reduction made absolutely no difference to the risk of stroke or heart attack. So, very much like the supposed link between cholesterol and heart disease (see Chapter 9), the theory of a link is looking pretty ordinary in the light of actual testing. Yes, vitamin B does change the level of a substance in our blood, but no, it doesn't affect heart-disease outcomes.

Vitamins C and E and heart disease

Vitamin C is also often touted as a cure for heart disease, but while it *is* an anti-oxidant, it's not used in the body to combat the oxidative stress that results in heart disease (see Chapter 10). Study after study has come up with a big fat zero, so while many marketing campaigns, particularly for orange juice, promote its anti-oxidant capabilities, the research has consistently shown that supplementing with vitamin C has no effect at all on heart-disease outcomes or death rates.

In the Physicians' Health Study reported in November 2008, 14 641 US doctors were followed for 10 years while they took either vitamin E or vitamin C supplements. Half the doctors were actually taking placebos instead, but neither they nor the folks assessing the results knew which was which. This double-blind, randomised nature of the trial, together with its large size and long duration, means that the evidence it produced is of very high quality. The results showed exactly no difference in the heart-disease outcomes for any of the groups. The vitamin E folks had just as many heart attacks as did the vitamin C folks, who in turn had just as many as the folks taking nothing. Even the 754 doctors distributed among the groups who'd previously suffered a heart attack showed no difference in outcome. The resounding conclusion is that while we certainly need vitamin E, we home-brew all we need, and shoving it in our mouths changes absolutely nothing (except the bank balance of the folks selling the supplement).

Other vitamin 'cures'

A recent suggestion is that vitamin K might help reduce osteoporosis in post-menopausal women, but a two-year randomised trial of 440 women published in 2008 concluded that high-dose vitamin K supplements had absolutely no effect on bone-mass density.

Multivitamins have not fared any better. A huge ongoing study involving 215 000 people in Hawaii and California released its 18-year report in 2011. It found a resounding nothing. The folks taking multivitamins did no better on any of the disease outcomes measured, which was just about everything you could think of. This is a questionnaire-based study, so it's not as strong as clinical trials, but it is very large and appears to confirm what most smaller studies say – the best that can be said about vitamin supplements is that they're mostly harmless.

Is folate good for everyone?

For most of us most of the time, taking vitamin supplements just means creating expensive urine. Our bodies are remarkably efficient at mining our incoming food supply for the stuff they need and chucking the rest. The theory has always been that if our vitamin stores are sitting at maximum (which they are for a lot of us a lot of the time), then any extras just get passed straight through. That's why we don't need a prescription to buy vitamins, why we can buy them in any grocery shop and why they're added willy-nilly to foods to make them 'healthy'. But some worrying research is starting to emerge that some vitamins could be very harmful if we take too much of them.

Folate and spina bifida

Folate has never been a public health problem in the West because it can be obtained in sufficient amounts from just about any grain-based food, most vegetables and most meats. But during the early 1990s, evidence emerged that neural tube defects in newborns (which occurred at a rate of around 4000 a year in the US and around 80 a year in Australia and included spina bifida) were related to whether the mother took folate supplements during pregnancy. Why this should be so isn't clear, because the mothers of children born with neural tube defects are not folate-deficient. Even more mysteriously, the problem persists for more than half the eventual births even if the mothers take the supplement.

The observed effect of folate supplementation was very real, and it clearly did prevent a significant percentage of neural tube defects. But folate only prevents neural tube defects if taken between the 21st and 27th day of pregnancy, a time when most women don't realise they're pregnant. This means that unless the mother was planning to become pregnant, she's unlikely to have been taking folate supplements at that crucial time. Since pregnant mothers need 50 per cent more folate than the rest of us, and because the consequences of a deficiency (for their babies and for them) are so very serious, a few countries have started fortifying foods with folates.

Spina bifida

Spina bifida (Latin for 'split spine'), is a birth defect caused by the incomplete closure of an embryo's neural tube (the brain and spinal cord), so that some vertebrae overlying the spinal cord are not fully formed and remain unfused and open. If the opening is large enough, this allows a portion of the spinal cord to protrude through the opening in the bones, which usually results in nerve damage causing at least some paralysis of the legs and affecting many organs and systems below the point of the 'split'. There's no cure. Treatments focus on the complications, and include surgery, medication and physiotherapy.

Is folate good for the rest of us?

Since the consequences of a folate deficiency are so very serious and many pregnancies are unplanned, in 1998 the US Government adopted a public health policy of fortifying all grain products with folic acid. Australia introduced similar mandatory fortification in September 2009. In the decade or so the US program has been running, it's reduced neural tube defects by about a quarter (from 4000 to 3000 per year), but folate consumption for the population as a whole has more than doubled. Now 38 per cent (up from 7 per cent) of older US adults have folate intakes above the recommended upper limit. Recent studies are suggesting this might turn out to be a significantly bigger health problem than neural tube defects.

Folate appears to be a double-edged sword when it comes to cancer. Having just enough folate (in combination with vitamin B12) protects DNA from replication errors that might lead to cancer. But once a cancer is established, folate is critical to the growth of tumours because it enables rapid cell reproduction, which is why it's so important during the early stages of pregnancy. This is not new news. The first anti-cancer drugs, successfully used in 1947 to induce remission in children with leukaemia, were in fact anti-folate drugs. When folic acid and vitamin B12 are in balance, they act together to protect us against anaemia by producing red blood cells and against cognitive decline, probably by protecting against DNA damage. But when folic acid is high and vitamin B12 is low, bad things happen.

A 2007 study of 1500 people over the age of 70 found that those with too little B12 and too much folic acid were four times more likely to develop anaemia and their risk of dementia increased from 18 to 45 per cent. But several large trials have recently concluded that getting to an age where dementia is a worry might be a lot harder if we're consuming too much folic acid in the first place. A 2006 study of post-menopausal women in Seattle revealed that in those who consumed more folic acid than the recommended amount (either because of its presence in supplemented food or because they took multivitamins containing it) the function of their natural killer T-cells, responsible for fighting infection and pre-cancerous cells, was reduced by 25 per cent. And a 10-year study of 25000 post-menopausal women found that those with the highest folic acid intake (from diet and supplements) had a 32 per cent increased risk of breast cancer compared to those on the lowest folate intake. Another study, also published in 2007, followed 1000 men and women for a decade after surgical treatment for colorectal cancer. Those taking folic acid supplements were at a significantly greater risk (52 per cent) of the cancer recurring than controls who were taking a placebo.

Food is now fortified with folate in Australia, New Zealand, South Africa, the United States, Canada and 47 other countries, largely in the Middle East, the Pacific Islands and the Caribbean. But no member or the European Union, including the UK, has done so, and debate still rages there about whether the potential benefits to newborns are outweighed by potential cancer risks to the rest of the population.

How harmful is vitamin A?

High levels of vitamin A from supplements but not food have been strongly associated with birth defects. A very large study of more than 22000 pregnant women, completed in 1995, found that around 1.5 per cent of them were taking vitamin A supplements that could cause serious defects in one in 57 births. It's now accepted medical advice that women shouldn't take vitamin A supplements or apply vitamin A–based skin creams during pregnancy. And if they're using prescribed versions of the creams to treat skin conditions such as psoriasis or acne, they should stop using them well before becoming pregnant. The creams contain a form of vitamin A called retinoids, which are very long-acting. Side effects and birth defects have been reported to occur months after discontinuing retinoid therapy.

High intakes of vitamin A supplements have also been strongly associated with osteoporosis. A study of 66000 Swedish women, published in 1998, revealed that the risk of hip fracture was doubled by a high intake of vitamin A supplements. But much like folate supplements, vitamin A supplements have also been associated with the possibility of increased cancer risk. One recent major randomised, placebo-controlled trial demonstrated a significant risk

of increased cancer rates among US smokers who were given vitamin A supplements.

Why don't vitamin supplements work?

Vitamin supplements have only really been part of the health message for the population at large since the 1970s, when Linus Pauling
started pushing them as a cure for everything. Thousands of trials
since have proved that self-medication with vitamin supplements
has absolutely no effect on your health, no matter how much you
spend on them. They also show that pregnant mothers need to take
folates if they're planning to become pregnant (stopping immediately after the birth) and shouldn't take vitamin A supplements or
use vitamin A skin creams when thinking about becoming pregnant or while pregnant. Quite a few of the larger trials have shown
increased risk of cancer for some supplements, but the doses used
in these trials were quite high, and studies of people taking supermarket vitamins have not shown similar risks.

The question that has dogged scientists during all four decades
of the vitamin-supplement craze is why don't they work? Studies in
which people have increased their vitamin intake by eating whole
foods (such as more vegetables) have consistently shown significant
benefits for heart-disease and cancer outcomes – about a 4 per cent
decline in risk for each additional daily portion of vegies. So why
doesn't a vitamin supplement produce the same result? Nobody
knows, but it's likely that the answer lies in the complexity of the
machine we wander around in.

Vitamins are not the only things in a stalk of broccoli or a
chunk of meat. There are thousands of chemical compounds swish-
ing around in our food. We know of and can name a few that we're
certain will cause serious disease if they're missing from our diet.
But in reality we have no idea how they interact with everything

else in the food supply or everything else in our body. It's incredibly arrogant of us to assume that we can pick out one substance from a whole food and consume just that to reap the same health benefits. But that's the assumption upon which the entire supplements industry has been built.

Our biochemical systems are extraordinarily complex. They make the inside of the most complex man-made machine (say, the laptop I'm writing this chapter on) look like a child's rattle. Yet we seem to assume we can just tinker with those systems based on very limited observations about what might or might not happen. It would be like me taking a hammer to my laptop because it was making a strange sound. My hammer might eliminate the sound, but it might just eliminate some other functions, too.

When we consume a vitamin from a whole food, we get it in its original packaging. Our body receives the vitamin and whatever else our metabolism is expecting in order to process it properly. We don't get too much of it because the food has just the amount we're designed to expect. We also take in any other substances (such as fibre and thousands of others) that might help regulate how much of the vitamin we absorb and even how much of it we can use. None of this happens when we take a supplement. Sure, an emergency dose of a supplement will cure a life-threatening deficiency (such as scurvy), but for most of us, most of the time, any extra is just a way to create expensive urine.

Should vitamins be added to food?

Rather than take a supplement, we can, with a little bit of knowledge, choose to get the vitamins we need from the foods in which they occur. But when supplementation enters the food supply, we have much less choice about what we're taking. Yes, we know that if we whack pregnant mothers with the folic acid hammer, some of their babies have significantly better outcomes. The critical point is that we don't know why this works, we just know it does. And based on that observation, our government has chosen to medicate the entire population. When we transfer that 'treatment' to all of us and decide we could all do with a whack with the same hammer, the effects may not be as benign as first thought. The US has been doing it for 10 years and the studies are starting to raise very real concerns. In Australia we've barely started – so I can't help wondering if we're going to be raising the same concerns in 10 years' time. The Brits are fearing to tread where Australians and Americans rush in. They're refusing to get the hammer out until they're sure it doesn't do any more damage than it fixes. Perhaps that's a more sensible path to tread.

But folic acid supplementation is not the greatest concern. The processed-food industry has created an entirely new category of foods stuffed to the brim with every supplement you could imagine. 'Functional foods' are the new growth industry – their sales are currently growing at five times the rate of normal food sales, and that growth is accelerating. Marketers have found that the best way to sell a bottle of sugar water to an increasingly sick and worried public is to tell them it contains twice their daily of allowance of – insert name of supplement du jour. Let's hope our bodies really are good at eliminating those excess supplements, or the science suggests we're in for a very rough ride indeed.

US functional food players ranked by 2008 sales. (*Source*: PWC)

Functional food players	Functional food brands
PepsiCo	Quaker Oats, Gatorade
Coca-Cola	Glaceau Vitaminwater, Odwalla juices
General Mills	Cheerios, Yoplait yoghurts

Kellogg's	Special K, Kashi cereals
Kraft	Capri Sun drinks, Balance Bar
Nestlé	Nesquik, PowerBar
Danone	Activia, Essensis
Unilever	Slim-fast, Blue Band
Yakult	Yakult

5. SALT AND OTHER MINERALS

Fat, carbohydrates, proteins and vitamins are all largely constructed from four basic building blocks: hydrogen, oxygen, nitrogen and carbon (the most important elements found in living things, along with a bit of sulfur). We pull the oxygen out of the air and get the other three from any plants we eat directly or indirectly (by eating an animal that ate a plant). We can make most of the complex chemicals we need out of these four basic units. Unfortunately, though, we do need a few extra chemicals to keep things running smoothly. These extras are what the nutritionists have labelled 'minerals' but how much of them we need varies widely. We need loads of some minerals (known as the bulk minerals) and very, very little of others (called the trace minerals). As an example, our body needs about 400 times more potassium (the bulk mineral we need the most of) than zinc (the trace mineral we need the most of).

The bulk minerals

Bulk mineral (from most to least required)	Major function	Best dietary sources
potassium	used (in combination with sodium) to run our electrical system (our brain, muscles and nerves)	pretty much any plant but especially leafy greens and vine-grown vegies
chlorine	used as part of the chemical process that turns food into energy	salt
sodium	Critical for transporting most things from outside a cell to the inside	salt
calcium	strengthening bones and teeth	milk
phosphorus	bone strength; part of chemical process that turns food into energy	milk
magnesium	bone strength; part of chemical process that turns food into energy	just about everything

It's almost completely impossible to be deficient in a bulk mineral, no matter what you eat. But a strict vegan will struggle to get enough calcium and phosphorus because absorption from soy milk and vegetable sources is not as efficient as from animal sources. It's totally impossible to be deficient in sodium and chlorine (the two parts of table salt) in Australia today, unless you knit your own food and grow your own underwear. Every processed food has salt added as a matter of course, particularly if the fat content has been lowered (salt and sugar are used to balance the taste and make up for the loss of the fat). We need salt and we need a fair bit of it (one to two teaspoons a day). It's vital for proper cellular function and in no way is it optional. We're also very good at getting rid of any salt we don't need, but for decades a controversy has raged about the dangers of · salt (see page 88 for more).

The remainder of the bulk minerals (calcium, phosphorus and, to a lesser extent, magnesium) are used primarily to keep our skeleton intact. They're critical to maintaining our bone mass, which in turn stops our bones from breaking easily. As we age, our capacity to store these minerals declines. Our bone mass increases sevenfold from birth to puberty and then triples from puberty to adulthood. It stays about the same until age 50 (for men) or menopause (for women) and then starts to decline at about 0.5–1 per cent a year. This eventually leads to osteoporosis (bone brittleness).

Calcium and vitamin D

We need sufficient vitamin D to absorb calcium and phosphorus from our food, so if we're not getting enough sun, we could be deficient in both of these minerals, no matter how much of them we consume. The supplements industry's answer is of course to sell us calcium (and sometimes phosphorus and magnesium) supplements or push products at us that are fortified with calcium (such as many of the more expensive milks). But the research once again suggests that our bodies are gonna do what they're gonna do, no matter how much we spend on supplements. Vitamin D and calcium supplements are often prescribed for older people at risk of suffering a fracture, but clinical trials have failed to prove that this has any effect whatsoever. One large recent trial in the UK gave 5292 people aged 70 or over high doses of calcium or vitamin D or both or a placebo for up to five years. There was absolutely no difference between any of the groups in bone density, falls, fractures, death or quality of life.

Because women lose 2–3 per cent of their bone mass during menopause, post-menopausal women are often encouraged to take supplements as well. A systematic review of 15 high-quality trials of this practice concluded in 2004 that at most this might result in the women losing 2 per cent less bone mass than they might otherwise. The longer the trial ran, the less difference there was, so perhaps the best that could be said was that the supplementation slightly slowed a process that happened anyway.

Is salt bad for us?

To most people's surprise at the time, salt reduction was included in the first (1977) edition of the *Dietary Goals for the United States*. The theory went that when we consume excessive amounts of salt, we overwhelm our kidneys' ability to remove it from our system. The excess salt then ends up in our bloodstream waiting to be cleared. While it's there it attracts water and this causes our blood volume (and therefore blood pressure) to increase. None of that's controversial. Excess salt *does* cause us to retain water until the kidneys can catch up and get rid of the extra salt and the extra water. The controversy is whether that transient effect amounts to a health problem.

What is blood pressure?

Blood pressure is the pressure our blood exerts on the walls of our blood vessels. During each heartbeat it varies between a maximum (systolic) and a minimum (diastolic) level. The further the blood vessel is from the heart, the less each of those pressures will be. Medically, blood pressure means the pressure as measured in the upper arm just above the elbow.

In Australia, normal adult blood pressure is defined as a systolic blood pressure of less than 120 mmHg and diastolic pressure of less than 80 mmHg (120/80 mmHg stated as '120 over 80'). If your numbers were higher than 140 over 90, you'd be diagnosed as having high blood pressure.

Some small salt studies have shown that decreasing dietary salt intake will lower blood pressure, but quite a few haven't. And the favourable results – a 3–4 per cent decrease for people with high blood pressure and 1–2 per cent for people with normal blood pressure – are hardly earth-shattering. In fact, it's possible to get similar effects just by decreasing the amount of water someone drinks before they have their blood pressure taken or by having a machine rather than a doctor take the blood pressure (around a quarter of us experience stress-related increases in blood pressure when confronted with doctors). And it doesn't take long to find major studies that flat-out contradict those results.

In 2008, a significant study showed that, at least in the US, low salt levels actually increase our risk of death from heart disease by about 80 per cent. And while the authors rather unconvincingly discounted that as a statistical anomaly, they concluded that salt intake was not a risk factor for heart disease or any other cause of death in the general population.

The most excellent way to raise blood pressure is to consume sugar. A by-product of sugar metabolism is the production of uric acid, and fructose is the only sugar that can raise uric acid levels (see Chapter 6 for more detail on this). Increased uric acid levels damage the kidneys and decrease our production of nitric oxide. We use nitric oxide to relax our arterial walls, so no nitric oxide means unrelaxed arteries and higher blood pressure. The uric acid accumulating in our kidneys over time starts to degrade kidney function. Damaged kidneys will ultimately be able to process salt less quickly, and that certainly won't help blood pressure. The studies clearly show that telling someone who has normal blood pressure not to eat salt is pointless. But if you already have high blood pressure, probably due to sugar consumption, then adding excess salt to the mix isn't going to help.

Are sports drinks good for us?

The vast majority of the bulk minerals we do eat (more than 95 per cent, including most of the salt) are passed back out again in our urine and sweat almost immediately. People who sweat a lot (by doing intense exercise for two or more hours at a time) will tend to lose some of these minerals (largely potassium and sodium) in their sweat and may need to replace those salts quickly if they don't want to feel weak and confused until their next meal. The same thing can happen after a severe bout of vomiting or diarrhoea or a heavy period. And this is why runners and people with the blurts and squirts are advised to take salt tablets. It's also the theoretical basis behind sports drinks.

In 1965, Dr Robert Cade, a kidney specialist, noticed that if he fed Gators a drink that mimicked human sweat they could play American football better than before. The Gators in question were his beloved University of Florida football team. American football in Florida requires very fit boys to run around, dressed in a spacesuit, in a climate similar to that of North Queensland for three hours at a time. As you might imagine, this took its toll on performance. The players were sweating up to 3 litres of fluid per hour, and while they could (and did) drink water, it diluted their sodium and potassium levels so much that their nerve and muscle function became temporarily impaired. Coaches routinely handed out salt tablets to combat this problem, but Dr Cade found that if he dissolved the salts in water, they were much more effective.

He also theorised that since fatigue was a very real problem for the players, it would be good to slip some instant energy into the drink. Cade chose to use glucose because that's the sugar we use for energy – our 'blood sugar' is glucose and most carbohydrates are eventually converted to glucose before we can burn them. He figured pure glucose would provide an instant energy boost, but there was just one wee problem with that 'solution' – it tasted a lot like, well, wee. The glucose was not sweet enough to overpower the taste of the salts, so he chucked in an artificial sweetener – and Gatorade was born. Unfortunately, Cade chose cyclamates as his sweetener just before the US Food and Drug Administration banned them. An urgent reformulation resulted in the glucose being replaced with sugar (sucrose).

Sugar was a less than ideal solution because it takes the body time to split it into its constituent fructose and glucose. Even worse, the fructose half impairs the uptake of the glucose. But hey, now it tasted great! And a great-tasting drink that could be legally sold was better than an ordinary drink containing a banned ingredient.

Gatorade, which is now owned by PepsiCo, has not looked back. It now controls 77 per cent of the $11 billion US sports drink market. Even Coke's Powerade is struggling to dent the Gatorade brand. Apparently, no self-respecting American athlete would be seen drinking anything else. Australians are less sensitive to the football heritage of Gatorade, so here the sports drink market is a practical duopoly, shared by Gatorade and Powerade. We still manage to put away more than 300 million bottles of sports drink every year, and the market is growing fast, so the big boys take their market share very seriously.

Both the major brands and their minor competitors are sweetened with sugar, and as a result are largely indistinguishable from the carbonated brethren dispensed from the mother ship. But the really ironic thing about sports drinks is that there's precious little science to suggest they're necessary at all. And any potential positive effects are enormously outweighed by the negative effects of consuming the sugar (see Chapter 6).

Whenever we exercise we need to drink water. If we exercise intensely and drink water for two and a half hours at a time, the water should contain some salts or we risk potentially fatal water intoxication. If we expect to be able to perform well for more than the first half-hour of strenuous exercise, then it would be a good idea to include some glucose in that water. Since very few of us meet the criteria for elite athletic performance (and I certainly don't), water will do just fine should we decide to don the lycra.

The trace minerals

The trace minerals: we don't need much of these but they are critical.

Trace mineral (from most to least required)	Major function	Best dietary sources
zinc	used in just about every chemical process; critically important for maintaining the structural integrity of proteins and switching genes on and off (particularly important for programmed cell death)	meat and fish
iron	formation of red blood cells	meat and fish
manganese	bone formation, cholesterol production and carbohydrate and fat metabolism	bread and tea
copper	connective tissue formation and iron metabolism	meat, fish and nuts
iodine	formation of thyroid hormones (which regulate our metabolic rate)	fish

selenium	assists with the formation of thyroid hormones	fish, chicken and eggs
molybdenum	assists in the metabolism of proteins	bread and nuts
chromium	increases insulin sensitivity	meat

We need very little of the trace minerals, but they're vitally important in keeping us functioning properly. And while we don't need much, some other things we eat can seriously affect our ability to absorb what we do need from our food. The amount of protein in our diet critically affects our ability to take in zinc, which binds to proteins.

Zinc

Even very small reductions in protein intake can have dramatic effects on the amount of zinc we absorb. In the Western world, the only people at risk of being zinc-deficient are vegetarians, who need to eat 50 per cent more zinc-containing foods (largely grains) to get equivalent amounts to meat-eaters. In the developing world, where diets have insufficient meat, zinc deficiency is a significant problem. Mild zinc deficiency can result in stunted growth, suboptimal pregnancy outcomes and impaired immune responses. Severe zinc deficiency can result not only in stunted growth but also alopaecia (baldness), diarrhoea, delayed sexual development (semen is a big consumer of zinc) and impotency, eye and skin lesions and impaired appetite.

Overconsumption of iron, copper and calcium can reduce our ability to absorb zinc (and chromium), while overconsumption of zinc can have the same effect on each of the others. This is particularly a problem for pregnant or breastfeeding women, who are often encouraged to take multivitamin tablets to guard against anaemia caused by iron deficiency. The excess iron in the supplements over-whelms the zinc-absorption system and can lead to zinc deficiency. We should only take iron supplements if we've been diagnosed as iron-deficient, which is extremely unlikely unless we're a pregnant vegetarian.

Iron

As for the rest of the trace minerals, we need very little iron. The iron we do have is held onto fiercely and we have no means of getting rid of any excess. We just top up our stores from our diet and then only as much as we need – the rest is simply ignored by our digestive system. Wholegrain cereals are often promoted as a source of iron, but we're largely unable to absorb it in that form. This means vegetarians have to work hard to get enough iron, but everybody else is extremely unlikely to be iron-deficient.

Chromium deficiency and sugar

Chromium is a controversial addition to the list of trace minerals, mainly because it's been claimed to help with just about everything, from depression to sexual performance, since the 1950s, when it was first identified in brewer's yeast. But trial after trial in humans has failed to bear out the often-patchy results from various animal studies. In the last three decades, however, it's become clear that chromium definitively plays a role in insulin sensitivity.

If we're deficient in chromium we become more resistant to insulin. It's almost impossible not to consume enough chromium if you live in Australia, and we get rid of most of the chromium we eat. Chromium deficiency is normally caused by the other side of the equation – excreting more than we should. Our chromium storage-management system can be messed up by – you guessed it – sugar. Sugar significantly affects the amount of chromium we

SALT AND OTHER MINERALS

eliminate. When we eat sugar, we excrete up to three times as much chromium as we normally would. This means that people consuming high amounts of sugar are likely to be chromium-deficient, and it's possible that this may lie behind, or at least play a part in, the development of insulin resistance in those people.

Iodine deficiency and fructose

Iodine is used by our thyroid gland to manufacture a couple of hormones with inconsiderately long names that have thankfully been abbreviated by the research community to T3 and T4. If a pregnant woman's thyroid gland can't get enough iodine to make these hormones, the consequences for her baby will be disastrous. Thyroid hormones are critical for the creation of the protective coating of nerves (a process called myelination), which is most active in the period from 22 weeks' gestation to just after birth. A range of recent studies show conclusively that even if the mother is only moderately iodine-deficient, the child will suffer a reduction in IQ of between 10 and 15 points. Severe iodine deficiency will result in significant mental retardation.

The research on iodine deficiency is well established, and is the driver behind the creation of 'iodised salt'. But in the last decade or so we've become a bit too good for plain old salt (rock salt only, please) and the alarm bells are starting to ring. Iodised salt now makes up less than 10 per cent of all salt sales. But even if you have a perfectly adequate amount of iodine in your diet, you may still be unable to produce enough of the thyroid hormones. And the best way to destroy your ability to absorb iodine (and most other trace minerals) is to consume a diet high in fructose.

A series of studies published in the 1980s by the US Department of Agriculture shows that fructose creates a copper deficiency. And a bit more research from Russia in the 1990s shows that a fructose-induced copper deficiency sharply decreases iodine hormone (T3 and T4) production by the thyroid gland. So even if there's plenty of iodine in a pregnant woman's diet, if that diet also includes plenty of fructose, she's playing Russian roulette with her child's IQ.

The combination of a high-fructose, low-iodine diet is starting to have a real impact on Australian women. A recent update to 2001 research from Westmead Hospital in Sydney suggests a 50 per cent increase in thyroid-hormone deficiencies in Australian pregnant mothers. The Australian Government's solution was exactly the same as its solution for neural tube defects. Since October 2009, all bread sold in Australia has included a dose of iodine. Now don't get me wrong, I don't know any mother who wouldn't give both her arms to ensure her baby had the best possible start in life, and as far as I can discern there's no downside to having too much iodine (since excess iodine is excreted in urine). But the research suggests that if we keep increasing the amount of fructose in our diet (see Chapter 6), then no matter how much iodine we put in our bread, pregnant mothers won't be able to convert it into the hormones they need.

Sugar isn't the only thing we can eat that affects our ability to use iodine. Some vegetables (cabbage, broccoli and Brussels sprouts) and soy contain substances called goitrogens, a class of chemicals that interfere with the production of thyroid hormones. This bit of news didn't strike my children as being particularly bad, until they discovered that cooking the vegies destroys the goitrogens, thereby making them perfectly good to eat. Soy is more problematic because only the fermented form (think miso and tempeh) is free from goitrogens. Unfermented soy, such as the kind you find in soy milk or tofu, is full of goitrogens and does impair our ability to use iodine.

Should we take mineral supplements?

The only way to be deficient in a bulk mineral is to avoid animal products, so vegans (particularly while pregnant) are at some risk of deficiencies in phosphorus and calcium. If they use soy products to overcome that problem, they'll struggle with potential iodine deficiency. With trace minerals, it's not so much what you eat to obtain the minerals (just about anything will do), it's what you eat *with* them that matters. Sugar, some raw vegies and soy affect the uptake of iodine. Sugar increases the loss of chromium, while overdosing on iron supplements (in fact, having any at all if you're not medically diagnosed as iron-deficient) will affect your uptake of copper, calcium and zinc. Unless you want to spend the rest of your life carefully adding up your dosages, it's probably best to avoid supplementation with trace minerals apart from eating the foods they come in. And it's probably an even better idea to delete sugar from your diet altogether.

PART 2

THE REAL CULPRITS: SUGAR AND POLYUNSATURATED FAT

Introduction

For the last three decades, Australians have been told that the cure for heart disease, diabetes and even cancer is to eat less saturated fat, eat less salt and lose weight by exercising. And we've listened. Low-fat foods dominate our supermarket shelves and we buy them. Between 1983 and 1995 the total fat consumed by the average Australian dropped 6 per cent. Manufacturers are constantly reducing the amount of saturated fat and sometimes even salt in our packaged foods. Meanwhile, organised exercise dominates our leisure time and our school time.

We're doing exactly what we're told to do and the statistics just keep getting worse. Between 1980 and 2000, the number of us who were obese more than doubled. Between 1990 and 2005, the number of Australians with diagnosed type 2 diabetes also more than doubled. Between 1985 and 2000, the rate of new prostate cancers increased by 15 per cent a year. Breast cancer increased by 37 per cent. And melanoma increased by 60 per cent in men and 22 per cent in women. There's only one possible explanation for why things have got so much worse in a period when we're clearly doing exactly what we're told to do – the advice is wrong.

This part of the book analyses the real causes of obesity, heart disease and cancer, which are just the tip of the iceberg. The basic message can be summarised in just two sentences. Sugar makes us fat and provides a perfect environment for the development of a list of chronic diseases we couldn't jump over even if sugar hadn't made us fat. Polyunsaturated seed oils give us heart disease (with the invaluable assistance of sugar) and cancer.

If you don't wish for any of those things in your or your loved ones' life, then all you need do is stop eating anything containing sugar (more specifically fructose) or polyunsaturated oils (more specifically seed oils). If you believe me without seeing the evidence, then skip to Part 3 and I'll talk you through how exactly you can eliminate fructose and seed oils from your diet. If you don't believe me (you untrusting sod, you), then keep reading the rest of Part 2.

6. WHY WE REALLY GAIN WEIGHT – SUGAR

No matter how special we'd like to think we are, when it comes to our body, we're just mammals. Okay, we're pretty bright mammals, but for all our braininess, the carcass we walk around in is 100 per cent pure mammal. Just like every other mammal, we have a sophisticated mechanism to make sure we keep functioning. When nutritionists first started guessing what made us fat, only one of the four major appetite-control hormones had been discovered. Then, it was almost acceptable to squeeze the square peg of a physics law into the round hole of human biochemistry. But those days are long gone, and so too should be our tolerance for that kind of guesswork. Now the science on appetite-control hormones is done, and it tells the real story of why and how we get fat. Fat, calories and carbohydrates in general are not the problem. Sugar, a particular type of carbohydrate, very much is.

The important sugars

Carbohydrates are broken down into simple sugars by our digestive system. There are only three important simple sugars: glucose, fructose and galactose. All of the other sugars you're likely to encounter in daily life are simply combinations of these three.

- **Glucose** is by far the most plentiful of the simple sugars. Pretty much every food except meat contains significant quantities of glucose. And our digestive system eventually converts even the protein in meat into glucose. It's a pretty important sugar to humans, as it's our primary fuel – no glucose means no us.
- **Galactose** is present in our environment in only very small quantities and is found mainly in dairy products in the form of lactose, where it's joined to a glucose molecule.
- **Fructose** is also relatively rare in nature. It's found primarily in ripe fruits, which is why it's sometimes call fruit sugar. Usually found together with glucose, it's what makes food taste sweet. As well as fruit, it's naturally present in honey (40 per cent), maple syrup (35 per cent) and agave syrup (90 per cent).
- **Sucrose** is what we think of when someone says 'table sugar'. It's immediately broken down by our body into one-half glucose and one-half fructose. Brown sugar, caster sugar, raw sugar, even low-GI sugar, are all just sucrose.

Our broken appetite-control system

When we eat fat and protein, our gut releases a hormone that tells us to stop eating when we've had enough. When we eat carbohydrates, our pancreas releases a different hormone that performs the same function.

But one carbohydrate doesn't trip either appetite-control switch – fructose. Fructose is one half of sugar, so everything that contains sugar contains fructose. That, on its own, wouldn't matter much if we didn't eat much fructose, in which case we'd just eat a few more calories than our brain thought we did. But our body doesn't just ignore the fructose. Our liver is blindingly efficient at converting it to fat. Before you even finish that apple juice or 'lite' yoghurt, the fructose in the first mouthful will be circulating in your bloodstream in the form of fats called triglycerides.

And that's nowhere near the worst of it. Researchers have also found that if you put that much fat in your arteries you mess up the appetite-control system for the foods that do trigger it.

A crash course in appetite-control hormones

There are four critical hormones in our appetite-control system:

1. **CCK**, which is released when we eat fat and protein. The more fat and protein we eat, the more CCK is released. An accumulation of CCK in our bloodstream signals to our appetite-control system that we've had enough to eat.

2. **Insulin**, which is released by our pancreas in response to the level of glucose in our bloodstream. This glucose is the direct end-product of eating all carbohydrates except fructose. As an appetite-control signal, insulin works in the same way as CCK.

3. **Leptin**, which is released by fat cells in our body. The more fat cells we have, the more leptin is released, so if everything's working fine, it acts as a kind of long-term fuel gauge for our appetite-control system. It works as an appetite suppressant in the same way as CCK and insulin, ensuring that our default appetite state is 'not hungry'.

4. **Ghrelin**, which is released by our stomach lining. It forces our intestine to contract, causing that bubbling, gurgling feeling, and reverses the effects of leptin. It acts as a temporary on-switch for our appetite-control system, stimulating our hunger.

When fat flows through our arteries, hormones such as insulin, CCK and leptin, which tell us when to stop eating, no longer work as well as they should. It's as if our appetite-control system is stuck at half-off. The hormonal signals telling us to stop eating can't cut through the noise from all that fat in our bloodstream. If we're not told to stop, we keep eating. So not only is fructose undetected and turned to fat, it actually increases the amount of other food we can eat. This is why, in the US for example, the average daily calorie intake has increased by 30 per cent in the last three decades.

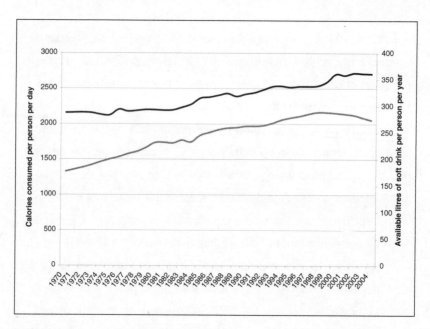

Calories consumed (*black*) versus soft drink available (*grey*) since 1970.

We keep our heart beating, our lungs pumping and our temperature stable on autopilot. We also ensure that our brain and every other cell in our body has exactly enough fuel to perform at its best, regardless of what's going on in the outside world. None of this requires a moment's thought. The control system for all of these and many other processes is our hormones. Hormones tell our bodies when and how much to grow. They tell women when to prepare for making babies. And they control how much fat we store and where we store it. We can't control our hormones with willpower or any other conscious thought. We can no more think ourselves taller or shorter than we can think ourselves a lower body temperature.

A child grows because hormones tell every relevant part of that child's body to grow. Some hormones instruct the cells to demand more energy and other hormones accommodate the demand by up-regulating appetite control. As a result, the child eats more and has the building blocks for growth. Growth drives appetite, not the other way round. A growing child can't fight hormone-driven appetite demands with willpower. And we can't control weight gain with willpower, either. Our appetite-control hormones are finely balanced to ensure we have just the right amount of energy on hand. Our hormones are so sophisticated they can even tell the difference between fat calories and calories from everything else (and adjust accordingly). But when that balance is disrupted, our fuel-management system can run seriously out of control. And a disrupted appetite-control system can cause the body to store too little or too much fuel.

Hormones, calories and diets

The first law of thermodynamics (see page 11) certainly says that when we gain weight there'll be an accompanying increase in the number of calories consumed or decrease in the number burned. In equations each side must equal the other, but that doesn't necessarily mean that increased calorie consumption *causes* the weight gain. It's equally logical to say that gaining weight is the driving force in the equation. In other words, weight gain *causes* us to consume more calories.

When a child grows they increase their body size and weight. These growth-hormone-driven changes cause the child to consume more calories, not the other way around. Not even the most rabid nutritionist would suggest that feeding a 10-year-old like an 18-year-old would help you get past those awkward teenage years more quickly. Growth happens because our hormone clock says it should. Calorie consumption just keeps up, so that the energy balance stays, well, balanced. We're perfectly happy to explain the equation that way when we talk about people who grow vertically. We're even happy to accept that pregnant women gain more weight than just the weight of the baby because hormones tell their bodies to fill the baby-pantry. Eating is the way we put on weight, it isn't the *reason* we put on weight. But for some reason, when Norm grows horizontally, nutritionists magically reverse the cause and effect, lurching from physics into psychiatry – and the cause suddenly becomes Norm's laziness or sloth (or both).

Obesity is a symptom of a failure in the balance of hormones controlling how much food we take in. This hormone dysfunction causes us to store too much fat in our cells, but because our body isn't aware the fat is there, it keeps demanding food. Our appetite-control system thinks we're starving, even while we have more than enough fat packed away (usually in very unsightly places). When an obese person restricts the amount of food they eat, they're not changing the underlying dysfunction in their appetite-control system. Their body thought it was starving before the diet, now it's really starving. It won't use its fat store to satisfy its need for food, because the hormonal disruption means it doesn't even know it's there. The hormones will force the body to sacrifice muscle and even organs to make up for the missing calories. And the whole time, the dieter will feel like they're starving to death. No wonder no one can stay on a diet!

The role of sugar

The science says sugar contains an appetite-hormone disruptor. With sugar in our diet, our bodies can no longer tell when we've had enough calories. Sugar gives our bodies permission to keep on eating, and we don't stop until we're physically restrained by the size of our stomach (or jeans). When that problem, well, passes, our broken appetite control gives us permission to keep eating until we're stuffed again. The result is that we're eating way too many calories, and fabulous as they are, our hormones can't read a calorie sticker slapped on a board at KFC.

Because all calories really measure is relative fat content, the processed-food industry isn't all that bothered about calorie labelling. They'll happily whack a calorie count on a can of soft drink full of appetite-hormone-disrupting sugar because they know it comes out looking pretty good next to an equivalent quantity of milk – 150 calories per 375 ml can of soft drink versus 240 calories for the same quantity of unflavoured milk. The sugar in the soft drink will make us want to eat more of everything, but milk, which actually fills us up, comes out looking sorry on a government-mandated calorie-counting sign. Sugar is effectively invisible on that sign. Indeed, they could even add more of the addictive substance and not materially affect the calorie count.

Once we understand that weight gain is caused by hormonal dysfunction, many previously mysterious things become clear. The failure of diets shouldn't come as a great surprise when we know how the human body deals with energy restriction. A diet that asks you, as all diets do, to consume fewer calories by exercising will-power is doomed to failure. Imagine how successful you'd be if you asked a child to exercise some willpower and stop growing! Fighting hormones with willpower is about as effective as paddling upstream with a barbed-wire oar. Diets, surgery and exercise do not affect the cause of weight gain – hormone dysfunction created by fructose – and so they don't work. Yet they remain the only targets of the billions spent 'combating' obesity in this country.

Obesity and chronic disease

Obesity is a symptom of appetite-control dysfunction, but it's not the only one. Heart disease, type 2 diabetes, kidney disease and dementia, to name just a few, are all symptoms of the same under-lying disorder. And, just like symptoms of any disease, the same symptoms don't appear for everybody at the same time. Not all kidney-disease sufferers are obese, although most are. Not all heart-disease victims are obese, although most are. And 15 per cent of American (and probably a similar percentage of Australian) type 2 diabetes sufferers are not overweight.

Type 2 diabetes

As we keep eating, the carbohydrates in our food are continually converted to blood sugar. Blood sugar keeps rising and we even-tually cannot produce enough insulin to remove the sugar from our bloodstream. Doctors describe that state as insulin resistance, the first stage of type 2 diabetes. Thirteen per cent of the US adult population is now suffering from type 2 diabetes. The equivalent number in 1965 was close to zero. When you add in those knock-ing on the door of the disease with insulin resistance, the number soars to 40 per cent of the population. As the graph shows, the fig-ures are similar for Australians.

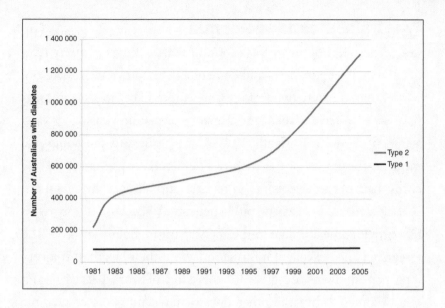

A recent study at the University of California persuaded 32 over-weight and obese people to try a 10-week diet that was either 25 per cent fructose or 25 per cent glucose. Both the glucose and the fructose were added to what the people normally ate, so that's a lot of extra sugar every day and you'd expect them all to gain weight. They all *did* put on weight as expected, but the people on the fructose diet ended up with 1.5 kilograms of new abdominal fat, whereas the people on the glucose diet did not. Abdominal fat has been shown to be a definitive sign of heart-attack risk, whereas fat stored in other places, such as the arms or legs, is not. The fructose group also had much higher levels of blood triglycerides, the circu-lating fats created by the fructose, which are a known predictor of heart disease. And they had 20 per cent higher insulin resistance, which is known to lead to type 2 diabetes.

Persistently high blood sugar is the most immediate effect of fruc-tose consumption. Eventually that leads to type 2 diabetes and other chronic diseases associated with high blood sugar, such as polycystic ovary syndrome, depression, anxiety and dementia, to name a few.

111

Type 2 diabetes and dementia

Researchers have known for a long time that there's a strong relationship between diabetes and dementia. Estimates have varied, but we're approximately two to four times more likely to have dementia if we also have diabetes or a history of insulin resistance. Now a bunch of Swedish identical twins are starting to put some real meat on the bones of the diabetes–dementia link. Almost 14 000 twins, part of the Swedish twin registry and all over the age of 65, participated in a recently published study. Because these twins had provided health data to the registry throughout their lives, the researchers had excellent information about their health over a very long period. Twins are great for this kind of work because when one becomes ill but the other doesn't, large numbers of possible causes can be eliminated as irrelevant. Clearly the twins share the same genetic make-up and they've usually been raised in an identical environment as well.

The Swedish study proved beyond any doubt that type 2 diabetes is associated with dementia, at least in Swedish twins. In fact, it concluded that we're 125 per cent more likely to develop dementia if we're diabetic. Even more interestingly, it showed that the longer we've had diabetes or insulin resistance, the more likely we are to develop dementia. In a somewhat depressing footnote, the researchers suggested that their estimate is probably a bit light-on because so many diabetics die before they're old enough to notice they're losing their grip.

A study of 2977 type 2 diabetes sufferers aged 55 and older, published a month after the twin study, took the issue further and established a direct link between sugar consumption and 'impaired cognitive function'. The subjects underwent a battery of tests that were part of a standardised set used to detect early signs of dementia. These tests are designed to measure such things as how fast

112

subjects perform calculations, how well they multitask and the accuracy of their memory.

The researchers compared the results of these tests to measures of each person's average blood-glucose levels over time. They found that the higher the blood-sugar level, the lower the score on all the tests. Just to put icing on the cake, the researchers noted that a 1 per cent rise in blood sugar takes you two whole years closer to dementia.

Kidney disease

Chronic kidney disease is now responsible for more than one in seven hospitalisations in Australia. Between 2001 and 2008, hospital admissions for kidney dialysis alone increased by 71 per cent. The news is even worse for Indigenous Australians. At the end of 2007, they were being treated for kidney disease at six times the rate of the rest of the Australian population. This is why the number of hospitalisations in the Northern Territory increased by an incredible 120 per cent between 2001 and 2008. The Territory has another interesting and perhaps dubious claim to fame: according to Coca-Cola, it has the highest per capita consumption of Coke in the world. Increasingly, the science is starting to suggest that this is more than a mere coincidence.

We don't know what causes most forms of chronic kidney disease and we certainly can't cure it, other than by replacing the kidneys. But a line of studies going back over half a century suggests that the cause and the cure might be linked to something called uric acid. Uric acid is a waste product created when we digest red meats. Genetic studies tell us that, uniquely among mammals, humans and great apes lost the ability to degrade uric acid about 60 million years ago, at the same time we lost the ability to make our own vitamin C (see Chapter 4). Our dogs can eat meat till the cows come home, but if we tried a trick like that we might be in a bit of trouble. Like most waste products circulating in our bloodstream, uric acid is removed from our body by our own little filtration system – the kidneys. Simply put, the theory goes that if we have too much uric acid, we end up clogging the filters in our kidneys and, over time, this degrades their capacity to work at all. Studies have shown that the theory is true for rats, but since rats process uric acid differently from us, the results can't be applied to humans.

In 2008, a major study conducted by the Medical University of Vienna went a long way to answering the question for humans. In that study 21 475 initially healthy subjects were tracked for seven years and their uric acid levels compared to the occurrence of kidney disease. The higher a person's uric acid levels, the higher their likelihood of developing kidney disease.

If the increased uric acid production observed in the general population was a result of eating meat, then we'd expect there to have been a steep increase in meat consumption over the last few decades. But our red meat consumption has been steadily falling since the 1970s. It turns out, though, that there's another truly excellent way to increase the amount of uric acid in a human's bloodstream – feed them sugar.

In 1989, the US Department of Agriculture's carbohydrate research team proved that they could cause a significant spike in uric acid levels just by feeding people fructose using a diet similar to one then consumed in the United States (with fructose as 20 per cent of calories). A much larger 2008 study of 4867 US schoolchildren found the same strong association between increased sugary-drink consumption and uric acid levels. And an analysis published in the same year used a similarly large database of results to link the consumption of sugary drinks with the onset of kidney disease in adults.

Uric acid is a by-product of the way our liver metabolises fructose. And unlike meat, fructose-consumption figures have gone nowhere but up for the last five decades. While all of that evidence is strongly persuasive, it isn't proof. No one has purposely fed a large group of people fructose to see how many died of kidney disease. But I rather suspect, sadly, that we're inadvertently conducting our own little experiment on the Indigenous population. Aboriginals and Torres Strait Islanders consume around twice as much sugary soft drink as the rest of us (although Australians in general are in the top 10 for per capita consumption in the world anyway). So it's no wonder that the Northern Territory, with its large Indigenous population, featured so prominently in Coke's statistics. And it's even less wonder, given what the science says about fructose, that it features so prominently in our kidney-disease statistics.

Kidney disease is massively debilitating. The only effective 'treatment' is getting hooked up to a dialysis machine three times a week. Meanwhile, the number of people needing that treatment is growing at the rate of 6 per cent every year. The only 'cure' is replacing the kidneys, if you're lucky enough to get to the head of the transplant queue (currently the wait is about four years) before you die. Kidney disease is now killing more Australians than either breast or prostate cancer, and more than twice as many as die on our roads every year.

Gout

The overproduction of uric acid is also known (uncontroversially) to be the cause of gout, a debilitating accumulation of uric acid in the joints that causes a form of arthritis. Back when folks ate much more meat and much less sugar, uric acid produced by overconsumption of red meat was the primary cause of gout, which was relatively rare. But the number of new cases of gout recorded in the

United States has doubled in the last two decades alone, and gout is now the most common form of inflammatory arthritis among American men. A 2007 study of 46393 US men, lasting 12 years, confirmed that the risk of developing gout was strongly associated with the consumption of sweetened soft drink (and therefore sugar). The men were divided into five groups according to their level of soft-drink consumption. The 20 per cent who consumed the most were 102 per cent more likely to be diagnosed with gout than the 20 per cent who consumed the least.

But wait, there's more. From the very moment it was first described in 1879, high blood pressure has been linked to gout and the level of uric acid in the bloodstream.

High blood pressure

Trial after trial conducted between 1972 and 2005 has shown that we're twice as likely to suffer from hypertension (high blood pressure) if we have high uric acid levels. Uric acid stops us producing a muscle relaxant called nitric oxide, and the theory goes that less nitric oxide means the smooth muscle cells of our arterial walls are less relaxed and therefore more constricted. This means that the diameter of our arteries is smaller than it might otherwise be, and our blood pressure is higher (as any plumber will tell you, a thinner pipe means higher pressure).

The reason for all the interest is that there are drugs (drug companies have much deeper pockets for this kind of research) that can be used to lower uric acid levels. Recent human trials have shown that those drugs do indeed lower blood pressure, but the evidence is clear that there's a much simpler preventative measure for all the conditions related to uric acid – kidney disease, gout and hypertension. Don't eat or drink sugar.

Diseases linked to fructose consumption so far	Diseases linked indirectly to fructose consumption
weight gain	sleep apnoea
type 2 diabetes	knee failure
polycystic ovary syndrome	depressed immune response
heart disease	cancer growth in general
stroke or aneurism	erectile dysfunction
high blood pressure	pancreatic cancer
gout	accelerated ageing
dementia	impaired muscle development
depression and anxiety	cretinism
fatty liver disease	varicose veins
cirrhosis of the liver	asthma
liver failure	ADD/ADHD
acute pancreatitis	
kidney disease	
tooth decay	

How fructose causes chronic disease

Enzymes control chemical reactions in our body. If we need a sugar (such as glucose or fructose) to be attached to a protein for some purpose, the appropriate enzyme will make sure that sugar gets attached to exactly the right part of the protein. The process of attachment is called glycosylation and we are only just beginning to understand the enormous array of uses our body has for glyco-sylated proteins, such as fending off disease and even inhibiting the development of type 2 diabetes. It is, however, possible for sugars to accidentally attach themselves to proteins without the help of an enzyme. When that happens, the process is called glycation, and it can result in sugars being attached in all sorts of unpredictable and haphazard ways.

Glycation occurs by accident and is really only likely to happen when our blood-sugar levels are high – the more sugar molecules floating around, the more likely some of them will crash into a protein. The good news is that in normal circumstances glycation is reversible. As soon as blood-sugar levels drop, most of the sugars and proteins will disengage and no harm is done. But if blood sugar stays high, as is the case for someone who is diabetic or pre-diabetic, the sugar–protein combo will undergo a series of reactions leading to the creation of an advanced glycation end-product (AGE).

Any sugar molecule can form AGEs, but glucose is the least reactive of all sugars. This is good, because it's the primary sugar in our bloodstream. The bad news is that the fructose half of sugar is 10 times more reactive than the glucose half. Eating sugar gives us a big shot of fructose and a big and immediate increase in AGE production. Making things much worse, fructose consumption also leads to an increase in insulin resistance. In the long term, the insulin resistance means our blood-glucose levels are persistently elevated. And this creates a second major source of AGEs.

If your doctor suspects you of being diabetic, they'll probably test your levels of HbA1c (or A1c for short). This test measures the level of a glycated form of haemoglobin (the protein that transports oxygen in your blood). A high A1c level indicates that there are significant amounts of AGEs in the blood. This is taken as a sure sign that your blood sugar is persistently too high. Our bodies are used to garden-variety (glucose-produced) AGEs, and we're pretty good at breaking them down and disposing of them. But even so, they accumulate in our organs and tissues over time and we, well, age (the acronym AGE was chosen very much on purpose). Unfortunately, the AGEs made with fructose molecules are resistant to our disposal system, so not only are they made at 10 times the rate, but they hang around like John Farnham on a comeback tour.

AGEs are junk. They're dangerous because they bond easily and randomly to each other and to other proteins in a process called cross-linking. AGEs accumulate pretty much everywhere in the body, but in some places they do much more damage than others. When they pile up in the lens, cornea and retina of the eye, they result in cataracts and macular degeneration, the leading cause of blindness in Australia. They also accumulate in the fine tubules of the kidneys and, combined with increased uric acid, result in loss of kidney function. They cross-link the collagen that otherwise gives our arterial walls and our skin their elasticity – hence the terms 'hardening' of the arteries and 'ageing' of the skin.

AGEs also accumulate in our brain. Brain cells ideally last a lifetime, which means they're much more likely to accumulate AGEs. When researchers start looking at the tangles of twisted proteins that accumulate in the brain cells of Alzheimer's patients, they discover AGEs in abundance. This is likely to be the reason why other researchers have picked up on the association between Alzheimer's (and other forms of dementia) and high blood sugar.

Fructose and cancer

Cancer is our biggest killer and sugar consumption has been in the frame as a cancer risk for a while now. In 2002, a study conducted by the US National Cancer Institute tried to find which food was most associated with pancreatic cancer, and the fructose half of sugar won first prize. The researchers identified 180 cases of pancreatic cancer from among 88 802 women who were monitored for 18 years as part of the Nurses' Health Study. Women who were overweight and sedentary with a high fructose intake had a 317 per cent greater chance of developing pancreatic cancer.

A 2006 study published by Sweden's Karolinska Institute demonstrated that the risk of developing pancreatic cancer was directly related to the amount of sugar in the diet. The people who said they drank soft drinks twice a day or more were 90 per cent more likely to develop pancreatic cancer than those who never drank them. Another study, published in February 2010, found that we're 87 per cent more likely to contract pancreatic cancer if we have two cans of soft drink a week (or about 10 grams of sugar a day on average).

These were all population studies, which are good for suggesting there may be a problem but give no clue as to the possible mechanism. In late 2010, a study from the University of California nailed down the likely reason. In the study, human pancreatic cancer cells were exposed to solutions of pure glucose and pure fructose in the lab. The researchers knew that consistently high blood-glucose levels (such as those occurring in a type 2 diabetic) will accelerate the growth of cancerous cells. They also knew that eating fructose directly increases levels of circulating fatty acids, which in turn reduces the effectiveness of insulin in clearing the blood of glucose. The persistently increased blood glucose leads to type 2 diabetes and feeds cancer. They tagged the glucose and fructose with radioactive carbon and found that the cancerous cells metabolised the fructose very differently from the glucose.

Cancer is out-of-control cellular reproduction. The fructose itself was being used by the cancer cells to create much more of the DNA and RNA that cells need in order to divide and proliferate. The difference between glucose and fructose appeared to be that, while both could be used for energy, only one supplied significant quantities of the building materials for tumour growth. A tumour treated with fructose grew much more aggressively than one in a bath of glucose. It appears from this study that lots of fructose in the diet creates a perfect environment for cancer growth. The persistently high blood glucose caused by the metabolism of fructose provides fuel and the fructose itself provides the material required for multiplication. What a perfect storm!

Studies of cells in a lab setting are not overly persuasive on their own. There are a lot of checks and balances in a living organism that simply do not exist when you isolate one type of cell. But these tests on pancreatic tumours combined with the strong line of population studies coming to pretty much the same conclusion are a powerful signal that fructose and cancer are strongly linked. In 2007, almost one in three Australian deaths (29 per cent) were caused by cancer. The incidence of breast cancer, the most common cancer among Australian women, has increased by 32 per cent in the last two decades. At the same time, the incidence of prostate cancer, the most common cancer among Australian men, has more than doubled. The studies don't tell us that fructose (and therefore sugar) causes cancer (we probably need to look to polyunsaturated fats for that – see Chapter 9), but they do tell us that, once cancer is established, fructose provides the perfect environment for its growth. Fructose is not an uninterested bystander in the development of cancer. Our renegade cells use it directly and significantly to accelerate their reproduction.

The bad news about sugar

Sugar makes us fat. It's directly converted to fat by our liver and it destroys our appetite control so we want to eat more of everything. The more sugar we eat, the fatter we'll be. The fructose half of sugar is a significant hormone disruptor and damages much more than our waistline. It throws our appetite regulation out of balance and convinces our body that it doesn't have any stored fat when there's more than enough to go around. But much worse than that, it causes significant disruption to important metabolic systems. The result of all that is clearly visible in the lengthening queues of people awaiting treatment for type 2 diabetes, chronic kidney disease, hypertension, cancer and dementia, among other chronic diseases.

We can't cure the powerful hormone disruption caused by fructose with willpower or exercise any more than by flapping our arms. But if we stop eating sugar we'll stop gaining weight. Even better, we'll start to lose weight dramatically and we'll do it without being on a diet. We'll still eat as much as we want of anything we want as long as it doesn't contain sugar. We won't feel restricted in any way and in fact we really won't feel like we're dieting at all – because we aren't. So let's put all the missteps in human nutrition over the last half-century behind us, admit we might have made a bit of a mistake and get down to eliminating the chemical cause of the problem – sugar (see Part 3 for how).

7. ALL ABOUT FATS

Before we dive headlong into the evidence on fats, it's worth taking a crash course in fat biochemistry. Biochemistry is never simple, so this section can get a little heavy at times. If you don't care about the details, move onto chapters 8–10.

What are fatty acids?

The building blocks of fats are called fatty acids. Fatty acids are chains of carbon atoms of varying lengths with hydrogen atoms along the sides and a carboxyl group (carbon, two oxygens and a hydrogen) at one end.

A chemical diagram of a fatty acid. C is carbon, H is hydrogen and O is oxygen; the double line in the carboxyl group on the right-hand side indicates a double bond – more about those below.

Saturated fatty acids

Each carbon atom in a fatty acid can potentially form four bonds with other atoms. In the picture below, the carbon atom at the left end has bonded with three hydrogen atoms and one carbon. The next one along has bonded with two carbon atoms and two hydrogen atoms.

Ignoring the carboxyl group at the right end, all of the carbon bonds in this fatty acid are occupied by another atom. In other words, the bonds are saturated. That's why this is called a saturated fatty acid.

$$H-\underset{\underset{H}{|}}{\overset{\overset{H}{|}}{C}}-\underset{\underset{H}{|}}{\overset{\overset{H}{|}}{C}}-\underset{\underset{H}{|}}{\overset{\overset{H}{|}}{C}}-\overset{\overset{O}{\diagup\diagup}}{C}\underset{O-H}{}$$

This is butyric acid, a short-chain (because there are only four carbon atoms) saturated fatty acid found in butter, parmesan cheese and vomit.

In a saturated fatty acid there are no bonds free for linking to anything else. Because all the atoms have a partner, they're very chemically stable molecules – it's very hard to get them to break their bonds and join up with other atoms or molecules.

Monounsaturated fatty acids

Sometimes, a fatty acid has two of its carbon atoms linked by two of the four available bonds. Because the molecule is no longer completely saturated with hydrogen, these types of fatty acid are called monounsaturated (for one double bond) fatty acids.

124

A monounsaturated fatty acid. This type of diagram assumes that there is a carbon atom at each peak and trough and two hydrogen atoms attached at that point. Nine carbons from the left end, there is a double bond and the carbon atoms on either side of it are attached to only one hydrogen rather than two. This is oleic acid, an omega-9 monounsaturated fat (the double bond is nine carbons from the left end) and the primary fat in olive oil.

Because double bonds are more electron-rich than single bonds, they are more reactive. This means that monounsaturated fatty acids are a little more chemically reactive than saturated fatty acids, but still not very reactive.

Our bodies can and do make both saturated fatty acids and monounsaturated fatty acids. There is, however, a class of fats we can't make – the polyunsaturated fats.

Polyunsaturated fatty acids

You might have guessed by now, but a polyunsaturated fatty acid is simply one with more than one double carbon–carbon bond.

Linoleic acid is an omega-6 polyunsaturated fat – the first of its two double bonds is six carbons from the left end of the chain. It's found in many seed oils, including grapeseed and sunflower oil.

Obviously, all those extra double carbon bonds make polyunsaturated fats the most reactive of all fatty acids. And the more double bonds they have – and most have quite a lot – the more reactive they are.

Why temperature matters

Fats and oils are simply different combinations of fatty acids. The more unsaturated fatty acids there are in the mix, the more likely the mixture is to be liquid at room temperature (22°C) and called an oil. The more saturated a fat, the more likely it is to be solid at room temperature and called a fat.

The more saturated fat there is in the mix, the less likely it is to react with air (or oxidise) and go rancid. Polyunsaturated fats oxidise quickly because they have a lot of double carbon bonds that can react with the oxygen in the air. This is why margarine will go rancid quickly if we leave it out of the fridge but butter could last for weeks or months, depending on the room temperature.

Mammals, including us, want their fat stores to be relatively liquid at their body temperature (around 37°C) and non-reactive. If our fat was as solid as candle wax, we wouldn't be able to move. In contrast, most seed-based fats (such as soy, canola and sunflower oil) need to be available to the plant when it's germinating (generally in the colder months), and so need to work at lower temperatures. Plants need fats that are higher in polyunsaturates and still liquid at lower temperatures. The same goes for fish, which need their fat to be liquid even in cold water.

Tropical plants have different concerns. They need their fat supplies not to go rancid in the tropical sun. So palm and coconut oils are very high in saturated fats.

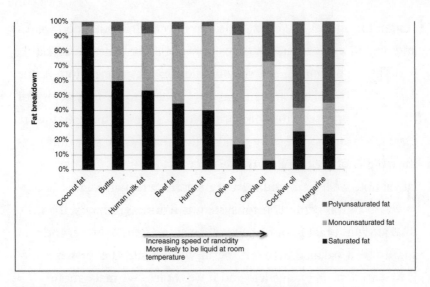

How fatty acids work in our body

In animals like us, fatty acids are stored in molecules called triglycerides (three fatty acids joined to a glycerol molecule, a relative of glucose). Triglycerides are too big to get through our cell membranes, so our digestive system splits them into their component parts and reassembles them once they've passed into the intestinal cells. The repackaged triglycerides then hit our blood supply and are transported to any cell that needs fatty acids. Imagine your body is a large city. Fatty acids are like supplies of timber for your city. The timber arrives on large ships, which equate to the food we eat. At the port, the ships must be unpacked and then the timber repacked onto delivery trucks to get it to where it needs to go in our city-body. Because fats cannot dissolve in our water-based bloodstream, they're carried by special delivery trucks, transport molecules called lipoproteins – more of them later, in Chapter 9.

The timber-fat that's being transported around our city-body comes in various lengths. It can be as short as four carbon atoms or as long as 24 carbon atoms. The shorter lengths are good for burning as fuel – short-chain fatty acids are an important energy-supply system for our cells. We can get them directly from the food we eat and we can make them ourselves from the carbohydrates we eat.

This is, of course, exactly where dietary fat comes from in the first place. The plants and animals we eat have made fatty acids (for their own purposes) from the carbohydrates they've made (if they're plants) or eaten (if they're animals). If we eat fat, we save ourselves the trouble of making it ourselves. But rest assured, whether we eat fat or not, we'll be manufacturing significant quantities of it ourselves. If our appetite-control system is working properly, then the total amount of fat in our body will be at the required level and will simply be a balance between the fat we eat and the fat we make. If we eat more, we make less and if we eat less we make more.

How we store fat

The cells unpack the triglyceride trucks that arrive at their loading bay and transport the individual fatty acids through the cell membrane into the cell. Using a process called oxidation, the cells chop up the shorter chain fatty acids to release their stored energy. If the cells don't happen to need energy at the moment, the fatty acids are repackaged as triglycerides and shipped off for storage in our fat cells.

Despite how permanent we might consider our wobbly fat stores to be, they're in constant motion. We have billions of cells constantly making chemical decisions about whether or not they need energy on a second-by-second basis. Billions of triglycerides are arriving at cell loading bays all over your body right now. Individual cells are deciding whether they need the cargo or whether it should be packed back up and sent for storage. Billions of stored triglycerides are constantly re-entering circulation from our fat-storage warehouses to ensure that any cell that decides it needs energy has plenty available.

Our fat-storage system is not a great big bucket to which we keep adding excess fat. It's more like a bucket with a hose in the top and a big hole in the bottom. If it fills faster than it empties, we accumulate stored fat and gain weight. If it empties faster than it fills, then fat storage decreases and we lose weight. Our fat-management system is a series of hormones. When everything is working fine, hormones tell us when we need to consume more food to top up the fat-storage warehouses and also tell us when we've got plenty of fat in storage.

We don't have a 'fat controller' running around checking on our fat supplies. Our monitoring system is much more elegant than that. Every single fat cell manufactures a hormone called leptin. The more fat cells we have, the more leptin is made.

Leptin is an appetite suppressant: the more fat we have in our warehouse, the stronger the appetite-suppressing signal. If everything is working fine, leptin acts as a magnificent auto-adjusting fuel gauge for our bodies. But this fuel gauge can be broken by the fructose half of sugar (see Chapter 6). When that happens we become leptin-resistant. This means our fuel gauge gives the body a false reading, constantly telling us we're on empty when we really have three-quarters of a tank. This means we keep stopping at the petrol station to fill 'er up.

Our cell membranes

We use fatty acids for much more than mere energy. Those triglyceride trucks backing up to the cell loading docks have more than just short-chain fatty acids on board. The longer chain fatty acids are the building materials for our cell membranes. They're the bigger timbers we use to construct the walls of the houses in our city-body. If we're healthy, the cell membrane of every cell in our body is largely constructed from saturated fatty acids, monounsaturated fatty acids and cholesterol. The fatty acids and the cholesterol give the cell membrane a flexible but strong structure.

Cholesterol is a critical part of the cell membrane. If our cells were houses and the cell membranes were the walls, the house frame would be the cholesterol and the cladding would be the fatty acids. The cholesterol provides the rigidity and the shape. Try building a house without a frame and you'd pretty quickly figure out what our cell membranes would be like without cholesterol.

In total, we need fatty acids for about half the molecules that make up our cell membranes. Saturated and monounsaturated fatty acids are nice straight molecules. They pack together well at the molecular level and make a cell-membrane surface that's both strong and flexible. But if the membrane were pure fat, it would be fairly solid and inflexible (think bacon fat at room temperature). So in the average cell membrane, cholesterol makes up the other half of the material in the membrane. This keeps the fatty acids apart and stops them crystallising into a solid. We need our cell membranes to be flexible and fluid, but not so fluid that they fall apart.

Our bodies work on the assumption that we'll have plenty of saturated and monounsaturated fats available for the important work of building cell membranes. But the proportion of saturated fat in our diet declined rapidly throughout most of the 20th century and has continued falling in the 21st century. The research that's accumulating suggests our bodies are not coping with that change.

8. GOOD FAT, (VERY) BAD FAT

The standard nutrition advice is that we should eat less animal fat, and most of us have taken that advice with gusto. That's why the supermarkets can get away with selling lean meat for twice the price of meat with the fat still attached. And it's why a 'healthy' margarine, stuffed to the brim with polyunsaturated vegetable oil, can be had for three or four times the price of ordinary old butter.

The 'eat less fat' message is dispensed by almost everyone who feels they can tell us what to eat. And it drives much of the front-of-pack 'healthy eating' labelling we see every day – 'light', 'low-fat' and '[insert percentage – preferably in the 90s]% fat-free' wink at us from every shelf.

The Australian Government's *Dietary Guidelines for Australians* are the gold standard for nutrition advice in this country. Dare to question the standard message not to eat animal fat and you'll eventually be directed back to those guidelines. They tell us to 'limit saturated fat and moderate total fat intake'. The reason is pretty obvious according to the writers. Eating fat makes us overweight. And because being overweight is a risk factor for type 2 diabetes, eating fat can be said to cause that as well.

According to the guidelines, dietary fat also causes coronary heart disease, but by a more convoluted route. Apparently, some of the fat we eat causes our cholesterol to rise. And since high cholesterol is a risk factor for heart disease, we should stop eating fat if we want to avoid that.

The only trouble with all of this is that it's just plain wrong. The evidence doesn't support any of the claims about fat. And it's becoming increasingly clear that the things we use to replace dietary animal fat (usually sugar and seed oils) are likely to be the real cause not just of heart disease, but also of type 2 diabetes, cancers and obesity.

Fat and heart disease

The biggest killers in Australia today are heart disease and stroke. Those diseases are largely attributable to a condition called atherosclerosis (from the Greek *athera*, meaning 'porridge' – because that's what it looks like – and *skleros*, meaning 'hard', leading to the rather descriptive 'arterial hardness caused by porridge'). In the popular imagination, the fat and cholesterol we eat sloshes around in our arteries. Given enough time, some of it will stick to our arterial walls. When enough of it sticks, it blocks off the arteries and bang – heart attack. It's a perception fanned by folks giving health advice, because it's easy to imagine and it helps keep us punters away from the 'bad' fats. It doesn't, however, have anything to do with the truth, and everyone involved in heart-disease research has always known that.

If you think about it for even a moment, it couldn't possibly work that way. Why would our largest blood vessels with the fastest moving blood, the ones nearest our heart, get 'clogged'? Surely in the clogging theory it would be the smallest veins with the slowest moving blood that clogged first? Atherosclerosis is actually the development of fat- and cholesterol-filled lesions inside the arterial wall – think big ugly pimple, but on the inside of an artery. When one of these lesions bursts, its contents spill into the artery and lead to heart attack or stroke. Researchers have been looking for the cause of the lesions for more than a century but we still don't know for sure. We don't know what causes them to rupture, either, and we certainly don't know what cholesterol has to do with it, if anything.

Cholesterol and atherosclerosis

We know that atherosclerotic lesions contain large amounts of cholesterol, but the body produces large amounts of cholesterol for use in cell membranes and hormone production anyway. The amount of cholesterol we consume in a day would be barely noticeable in the sea of cholesterol our body produces. The body adjusts how much it makes to take account of what we eat – it won't bother making any if we decide to pick some up for free from our food. Our internal cholesterol-feedback systems can't tell the difference between the cholesterol we make and the cholesterol we eat, so the question has always been whether eating cholesterol results in any worse atherosclerosis than not eating it.

Unfortunately, blood cholesterol was one of the very first blood tests developed (in 1934). In the 1930s there weren't many things a doctor could measure in a blood sample, but cholesterol was one of them. When the only tool you have is a hammer, everything starts to look like a nail. And when the only measurement you can take is cholesterol, to heart-disease researchers everything looked like it could be cured by reducing cholesterol.

The idea that eating cholesterol might lead to atherosclerosis really started with a rabbit. A bunch of Russian rabbits, to be more precise. The bunnies in question were the unfortunate subjects of some experiments done in 1913 by Nikolai Anitschkow, a young experimental pathologist working at the Military Medical Academy in St Petersburg.

Anitschkow was trying to reproduce human-like arterial lesions in animals. He theorised that the lesions formed in response to inflammation or injury in the arterial wall, in much the same way a scar forms when we cut our skin. But animal experiments in the first decades of the 20th century had failed to produce the expected results: mechanical injury to blood vessels didn't work; increasing blood pressure didn't work; severing or irritating nerves didn't work; and even injecting salt or toxins didn't produce the lesions.

Another researcher in Anitschkow's laboratory managed to do it, however, by feeding the rabbits meat, cheese and eggs. Anitschkow, assigned to find out what part of that diet actually caused the lesions, eventually discovered that if he fed the rabbits purified cholesterol from egg yolks dissolved in sunflower oil, they developed lesions that looked a lot like the atherosclerosis found in human sufferers of heart disease. The rabbits never had heart attacks, though, because their lesions never burst. Control bunnies fed just the sunflower oil didn't develop the lesions.

The research didn't exactly make a splash at the time. It was largely ignored because no one could reproduce the results in animals that weren't herbivores. A rabbit's normal diet includes exactly zero cholesterol. They don't eat steak or eggs (even chocolate ones, which might suggest why the Easter Bunny is a trustworthy courier). Even Anitschkow failed to get a result in dogs, which are natural carnivores. No matter how much cholesterol he fed them, he couldn't produce lesions. He decided that carnivores must have evolved a protective mechanism that was unnecessary in herbivores. This, of course, meant that omnivores like us, with a decided preference for meat when we can get it, were probably protected as well, and the research was most likely irrelevant to humans.

In 1946, a leading medical textbook summarised the accepted view on cholesterol by saying that, while there was absolutely no doubt that cholesterol and fat deposits are part of atherosclerosis, there was no evidence that high blood cholesterol had anything much to do with it. By 1950, the theory that diet was at all associated with cholesterol levels was six feet under as far as the research community was concerned. *Circulation*, the journal of the American Heart Association, had just published the first detailed human study of cholesterol levels in heart-attack patients. The study compared the diet and blood cholesterol of 90 American men who'd suffered heart attacks at ages less than 40 with those of 130 healthy American men. The researchers found absolutely no relationship between the amount of cholesterol a subject ate and their blood-cholesterol reading. There was also no difference between the amount of cholesterol consumed by the heart-attack sufferers and the healthy patients. The 'cholesterol gives you heart disease' message was all but dead, but it was about to be revived from an unlikely quarter.

Ancel Keys, cholesterol and heart disease

In 1939, Ancel Keys, a 31-year-old marine biologist, joined the Mayo Foundation, run by the University of Minnesota in Rochester, Minnesota, where he created the Division of Human Physiology and Biochemistry. The following year he was invited to organise what was to become the Laboratory of Physiological Hygiene at the university's main campus in Minneapolis. By this time, World War II was engulfing Europe, and America's involvement was becoming more certain by the day. The US Department of Defense was one of the biggest paying customers of Keys's new lab, and one of his first contracts was to run subsistence tests for the department.

The Defense Department had to keep an eye on its budget, so Keys's first major assignment was to determine the least amount of food required to keep a combat soldier alive and in fighting condition. The Army wanted a complete meal small enough to fit into a soldier's pocket, so Keys and his team scoured the local shops to create what was essentially a lunchbox full of high-calorie, long-life foods. Each waterproof box contained a tin of meat or cheese, biscuits, a chocolate bar and hard candy, coffee, soup powder, chewing gum, toilet paper and, of course, cigarettes. The infamous K-rations ('K' for Keys) became – and remain, albeit heavily modified – a staple of the US military. Overnight, Ancel Keys became one of the first ever experts in human nutrition. By 1941, he was special assistant to the Secretary of War.

The starvation studies Keys carried out on conscientious objectors during the war (see Chapter 1) gave him access to significant government population health and food data coming out of post-war Europe. Looking at these data, Keys noticed that, as food supplies reached starvation levels, the death rate from coronary heart disease dropped significantly. He couldn't explain that counterintuitive observation – surely more people should be dying of heart attacks as they starved, not fewer.

Keys developed a theory to explain the data. He thought that a full-calorie diet contained more animal products and fat and therefore more cholesterol than a starvation diet. He knew of Anitschkow's experiments and theorised that, just as with rabbits, if there's too much cholesterol in the blood of well-fed Europeans, it can accumulate and cause atherosclerosis, and this could lead to heart attack or stroke. Starving people reduced their fat (and therefore cholesterol) intake, and had fewer heart attacks.

Keys's research into heart disease

Post-war America was by then in the grip of an epidemic of heart disease. In 1925, only 20 men per 100000 aged 45–54 died of heart disease. By 1950, 10 times that number were dying. For men aged 55–64, the increase was even more pronounced, jumping from about 40 per 100000 in 1925 to almost 600 per 100000 by 1950. Keys believed he'd nutted out why these well-fed middle-aged men were dying. They were all eating too much fat, while people on the starvation diet had less heart disease because they'd eliminated fat.

Keys's theorised correlation between dietary fat, cholesterol and heart disease was just a theory, and it was based on just a few observations. But he was, by then, a very influential researcher. Dr Keys proposed a study that would follow a large number of apparently healthy middle-aged executives for many years, comparing the characteristics of those who had heart attacks along the way with those who didn't. He obtained funding for this long-range study of the factors involved in what he called 'degeneration of the heart', recruited 286 Minnesota businessmen and set up a metabolic research unit at a local hospital.

As Keys expected, heart disease was the most frequent cause of death, and the most common risk factor was smoking (which is ironic, given the K-ration included cigarettes). Keys identified blood pressure and blood cholesterol as other risk factors for heart attack or death. But even before this study began providing answers, he was designing a bigger and better study. In 1953, he published a pilot study comparing fat consumption with deaths from heart disease in Japan, Italy, England and Wales, Australia, Canada and the US (see the graph over the page). He chose those countries from a database of 22 countries, but he didn't say why he selected those particular countries.

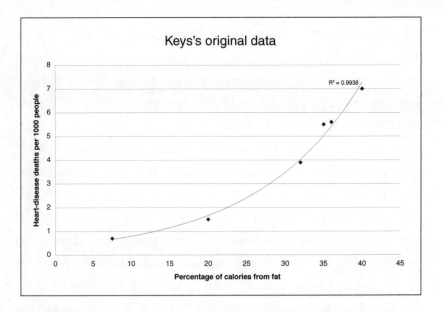

Keys's original data

$R^2 = 0.9938$

Heart-disease deaths per 1000 people

Percentage of calories from fat

Keys showed an almost perfect correlation between heart-disease deaths and the amount of fat in the diet. R^2 is a measure of correlation. An R^2 of 1 would be a perfect correlation.

While the countries he chose certainly demonstrated a very strong (almost perfect) correlation between heart-disease deaths and the amount of fat in the diet, it very quickly became clear that choosing a different set of countries would have yielded a very different result. If, for example, he'd chosen Israel, Austria, Switzerland, Germany, the Netherlands and Norway (see graph opposite), he'd have been able to suggest that eating fat *reduces* our risk of heart disease! If data points from the 15 countries Dr Keys failed to include are added to his graph, there's still a weak correlation – $R^2 = 0.39$ – but the correlation is far less convincing and it's much more difficult to maintain that there's any relationship between dietary-fat consumption and heart disease. As several researchers pointed out at the time, he could just as easily have shown a correlation between protein consumption and heart disease (and lobbied for a nut-free vegetarian diet, presumably).

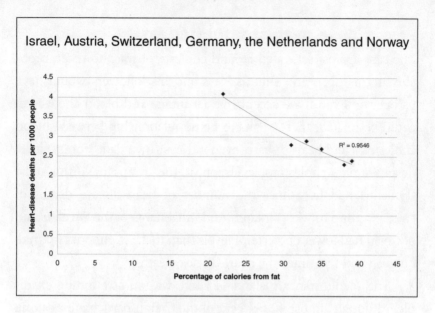

Israel, Austria, Switzerland, Germany, the Netherlands and Norway

What Keys's graph would have looked like had he chosen six other countries. This suggests a strong inverse correlation between fat and heart disease – the more fat you eat, the less likely you are to have a heart attack.

The purpose of Keys's pilot study was to talk the US Government into funding his more elaborate 'seven-countries study'. And it worked. How could a Congressman ignore such a strong correlation? The study, which launched in 1958 and ran for the following decade, enrolled 12 763 men aged 40–59 in 16 groups from seven countries. The now-famous study seemed to show that the higher the level of fat in a nation's diet, the higher its citizens' average blood-cholesterol readings and the higher the number of deaths from coronary heart disease.

Keys explained these results by suggesting that a diet rich in the saturated fats found in animal products such as meat, eggs and dairy foods produces higher levels of blood cholesterol, and that this, in turn, increases the risk of atherosclerosis and results in heart attacks.

Keys's 'case' against saturated fat

The case against saturated fat and cholesterol was, however, probably not as open and shut as Keys and his followers would have us believe. Even if we accept that fat intake and blood cholesterol could be related, there seems to be no relationship between blood cholesterol and heart disease, even in Keys's own data. For instance, despite similar cholesterol levels, one of the groups in North Karelia (Finland) had five times the number of heart-disease deaths of another group in west Finland. And inhabitants of the Greek island of Corfu had lower cholesterol levels than their neighbours in Crete but also had five times the heart-disease deaths.

The Mediterranean island of Crete was an astounding example. Although almost 40 per cent of the Cretan participants' calorie intake came from fat, they experienced the lowest death rates of all countries studied. Subsequent studies have also found enormous variations in heart-disease rates within countries, despite comparable blood-cholesterol levels.

Keys explained these aberrations by theorising that the majority of the fat in the Cretan diet came from olive oil and fish, which are rich in unsaturated fats, unlike the American and Finnish diets (although he presumably meant just the diet of the Fins in North Karelia), which are high in saturated animal fats. He concluded that although saturated fat can be harmful to your health, unsaturated fats can have positive health benefits.

What's really in animal and vegetable fats

Ancel Keys equated animal fats with saturated fats and vegetable oils with unsaturated fats, and his message has stayed with us. But the reality is that neither statement is true. Animal fats and vegetable oils both include unsaturated and saturated fats.

> Butter is 51 per cent saturated fat and 24 per cent unsaturated fat. Olive oil is 14 per cent saturated and 84 per cent unsaturated, but coconut oil (another vegetable fat) is 90 per cent saturated. So while it's true to suggest that most vegetable oils have more unsaturated fat than animal fats, it isn't true to say that animal fat is entirely saturated and plant fat is entirely unsaturated.

Keys and the 'Mediterranean diet'

Keys aggressively promoted his theory linking heart disease with a diet high in saturated fats. With his wife and former lab assistant Margaret, he popularised the 'Mediterranean diet' in a series of best-selling books (starting with *Eat Well and Stay Well*, first published in 1959). The diet is based on mimicking the food intake of the Mediterranean cultures that scored well in his seven-countries study. It suggested we eat low levels of meat and dairy to avoid saturated fats but to get loads of unsaturated fats by eating plenty of olive oil and fish. It also allowed us three to four eggs a week, as many vegetables, fruit and nuts as we could eat, and one to two glasses of wine or beer a day. The Mediterranean diet is quite high in salt, as foods such as olives, salt-cured cheeses, anchovies, capers, salted fish roe, and salads dressed with olive oil all contain high levels of salt, but at that time the paranoia about dietary salt (see Chapter 5) was yet to be stirred up.

Keys was almost evangelical in his belief that all Americans should be eating a diet like that consumed in the Mediterranean. When a group of Scandinavian medical associations published the first ever guide to public nutrition in 1968, Keys made sure it was translated and published in a major American journal within four months. *Medicinska synpunkter på folkkosten i de Nordiska länderna* (*Medical Viewpoints on People's Food in the Scandinavian Countries*) cited Keys's work favourably, recommending a reduced intake of total fat and saturated fat and an increase in polyunsaturated fat in order to reduce heart disease.

There was nothing like the Scandinavian guidelines in the United States or anywhere else, so Keys lobbied long and hard in favour of them being published in English. And he was not without support. Based on his work and some other very small hospital-based trials, as early as 1961 the American Heart Association had already accepted what it called 'the causal relationship between dietary fat and heart disease' and recommended, in guidelines co-authored by Ancel Keys, that doctors advise people at high risk of heart attack to modify their diet. The suggested modification was to substitute polyunsaturated vegetable oils for saturated animal fats.

By 1964, the Heart Association had extended its dietary rec-ommendations, without any change in the available evidence, to include the general public rather than just those at high risk of heart attack. In 1965, the American Medical Association published similar recommendations, and by 1971, the Australian Heart Foundation did the same, although at first restricting its advice to patients with high blood cholesterol.

The first national guidelines for the US, *Dietary Goals for the United States*, were released in 1977, published by the US Senate's Select Committee on Nutrition and Human Needs. The guidelines merged Keys's saturated-fat hypothesis with the salt-hypertension hypothesis, which had received barely any attention until that point (see Chapter 5). The publication took most people in the nutri-tion community completely by surprise, not least because there was almost no evidence to support many of its recommendations.

None of this stopped the goals being widely copied with little apparent independent thought. In 1979, the Australian Department of Health and the Dietitians Association of Australia published identical dietary guidelines advising us to 'avoid eating too much fat' and eat more 'breads and cereals'. Even so, the public remained blissfully unaware of the news on fat. Very few doctors paid any attention to cholesterol, and dietary advice was almost non-existent.

The role of drug companies

Then the drug companies, which had been working on cholesterol-lowering medication, came through with some hard evidence. The Lipid Research Clinics Coronary Primary Prevention Trial had been testing the effect of a cholesterol-lowering drug since 1977, when the *Dietary Goals for the United States* first came out. All trial subjects were placed on a low-cholesterol, low-saturated fat diet and trained in how to select these types of food.

The only difference between the two trial groups was that one was taking a cholesterol-lowering drug and the other was taking a placebo. The results were big news at the time. The drug apparently reduced cholesterol by 8.5 per cent, and the study showed that 2 per cent of the men in the placebo group but just 1.6 per cent of the men in the treatment group died from heart disease over the eight-year course of the study. The difference wasn't terribly impressive, but it was a result for believers that cholesterol kills us – if they squinted and looked at the statistics just the right way. One less publicised aspect of the study was that deaths from cancer increased in the group taking the cholesterol-lowering drugs, so the overall death rate in the two groups was the same.

Since both groups were on exactly the same diet, the trial wasn't a dietary trial but a drug trial. Nevertheless, the US Heart Foundation and National Institutes of Health decided to take a leap of faith and believe that anything that lowered cholesterol must also lower heart-disease death rates. They concluded that if people could be motivated to consume less saturated fat, it would lower their cholesterol. And if they could lower their cholesterol, they'd lower their risk of death from heart disease.

Government dietary guidelines

The result was the release in 1980 of the first ever dietary guidelines for the United States, jointly produced by the US Department of Health and the US Department of Agriculture. Guideline number 3 of six was to 'Avoid too much fat, saturated fat and cholesterol'. The reasoning was clear and simple. Eating too much saturated fat and cholesterol can increase your blood-cholesterol level – which is perfectly true – and high blood cholesterol increases your risk of heart attack – which was a great big guess. The guidelines suggested that Americans choose lean meat, fish, poultry and dried beans for protein, limit their consumption of eggs, butter, cream, hydrogen-ated margarines, shortenings and coconut oil, trim excess fat off meat, and boil rather than fry their food.

Hot on the heels of these dietary guidelines came America's most extensive public-relations campaign about any health issue. The aim was to convince the nutrition profession as well as the public that avoiding dietary fat was a key element in the prevention and treatment of heart disease. The US National Institute of Health, the American Heart Association, the US Department of Agriculture, a host of medical organisations and the processed-food industry promoted this concept until they were hoarse.

By 1981, Australia had copied the US guidelines and produced its own national dietary guidelines. The Department of Health had published guides on what to eat since 1954, but rather than attempt to improve us, these had focused on the nutrients we need just to stay alive. The new guidelines were different. For the first time they were aimed at preventing chronic diseases. Fat was blamed for the increasing rates of heart disease, so our guidelines recommended we should 'avoid eating too much fat'. And that's pretty much what the guidelines have said since then. In short, the message is that saturated fat and dietary cholesterol give you heart disease so you should eat a lot less of them.

I very much doubt that anyone actually pores over the guidelines while they fill their shopping trolley, but many of us use them without realising it. They're the basis for the daily-intake recommendations on every packaged food we buy. They form the foundation for every piece of advice any government agency or nutritionist gives us, from school canteens to hospitals. And every meal for our military forces and hospital patients is created using a policy based on those guidelines. Any time a meal claims to be 'nutritious' or 'balanced', that means it's compliant with those guidelines. They affect what we eat in many subtle ways, without most of us being aware they exist at all.

The cascade from dubious rabbit study, to selective international study, to dietary goal for high-risk groups, to national guidelines for everyone, to a '99 per cent fat-free' label on everything is now complete. As we approach the 100th anniversary of the meat-fed bunny's death (at the hands of a lab technician, not heart disease), the evidence is persistently failing to materialise, even though it should have been found before governments issued mass dietary advice. Indeed the evidence now tells us Keys guessed wrong, the American Heart Association backed the wrong pony and our lot – the Australian Heart Foundation – trailed along after them, blissfully unaware.

The truth about saturated fat

So far the vast majority of high-quality observational studies have found no connection whatsoever between saturated-fat consumption and heart-attack risk. The studies considered the most reliable are known as prospective studies.

Keys's study was an epidemiological or population study, and one of the persistent criticisms of his work was that it compared diverse populations. Comparing particular populations (men) from a very select group of countries seemed to ensure that multiple factors besides diet, such as genetics, smoking rates and the availability of healthcare, could significantly influence any outcome. Even worse, those population groups might not have been representative of their national population at all.

In a prospective study, however, investigators find a group of initially healthy people, record information about them – in this case what they eat, what they've eaten in the past and their vital statistics – and watch who gets sick over the years. A prospective study allows the researchers to drill down into the details with a known set of individuals.

One of the earliest prospective attempts to figure out whether dietary-fat consumption could have an effect on our risk of death by heart attack was the Framingham Heart Study, established by the US Government in 1948 to try to explain the rising tide of heart-disease-related deaths. The researchers recruited 5209 men and women aged 30–62 from the town of Framingham, Massachusetts. Every two years, the subjects gave a detailed medical history, and underwent a physical examination and laboratory tests.

In 1960, the Framingham Heart Study was the first to publish strong evidence that smoking increases the risk of heart disease. But its results on the dietary-fat front have been far less conclusive. The study continues to this day, but it's so far failed to show any correlation between the amount or type of fat consumed and heart-disease risk. It's also failed to show any relationship between high blood-cholesterol levels and increased heart-disease risk.

If anything, the relationship is the opposite of what Keys would have predicted. Dr William Castelli, the director of the study from

1979 to 1995, famously said in 1992: 'in Framingham . . . the more saturated fat one ate, the more cholesterol one ate, the more calories one ate, the lower the person's [blood] cholesterol . . . we found that the people who ate the most cholesterol, ate the most saturated fat, ate the most calories, weighed the least and were the most physically active.'

But before any results were available from Framingham, another major prospective study commenced in 1957 at the Western Electric Company in Chicago. In that study, 1989 men aged 40–55 were randomly selected from a 20 000-strong workforce. They were chosen on the basis that they had no symptoms of heart disease when the study started. The men were not told anything about what they should or shouldn't be eating, they simply attended a medical examination once a year for five years and filled in surveys about what they ate. By the end of the study, 88 cases of heart disease had developed. The researchers found that there was an increased chance of developing heart disease if the patient had persistently high blood cholesterol, but they couldn't find any association between what a person ate or their weight and their blood cholesterol. So perhaps cholesterol was implicated in heart disease, but neither blood cholesterol nor the men's chance of suffering a heart attack seemed to be affected by what they ate.

The Honolulu Heart Study, as it became known, was the next major study to look at the factors in heart health. It assessed the health of 7705 men aged 45–68, all of Japanese ancestry and living in Hawaii. The men were followed up over a six-year period that ended in 1978. The study suggested that men who ate fewer carbohydrate foods (bread, rice, pasta) and drank less alcohol were less likely develop heart disease. But there was absolutely no evidence that dietary-fat consumption or dietary-cholesterol consumption made any difference whatsoever.

The Framingham, Western Electric and Honolulu study results were all available before the release of the 1980 *Dietary Guidelines for Americans* (and the 1981 Australian guidelines), but by then the momentum behind the 'eat less fat' message had built to such an extent that it was too late to put the toothpaste back in the tube. The fine print in the US guidelines acknowledged that some people can eat a diet high in saturated fat and cholesterol but still have normal blood cholesterol, while some people have high blood cholesterol even though they eat a low-fat diet – which to me reads like a weather forecast that predicts rain as long as it's not sunny. But this didn't stop the guidelines making the headline recommendation to eat 'less saturated fat'.

Since the 1980s, study after study has collectively followed hundreds of thousands of people, initially men and then women. And study after study has come to exactly the same conclusion. In 2001, a systematic review in the *British Medical Journal* of all major studies published to that point concluded that there was no decisive evidence that that amount or type of fat we eat has any effect on our chances of developing or dying from heart disease or stroke. And the hits keep coming.

The most recently completed prospective study, the 2005 Malmö Diet and Cancer Study, perhaps put it best when it concluded, after observing 28 098 middle-aged people for five years, that the guidelines were wrong: 'individuals receiving more than 30 per cent of their total daily energy from fat and more than 10 per cent from saturated fat, did not have increased [death rates]. Current dietary guidelines concerning fat intake are thus generally not supported by our observational results.' The translation of that is: 'The dietary guidelines are wrong, wrong, WRONG!'

The power of marketing

The complete lack of evidence has not, however, stopped the marketing machine behind the 'don't eat saturated fat' message. Once the message went public, important reputations were built on it being true. When the US Government and the American Heart Association started putting the case against saturated fat in the early 1980s, the public paid attention. People stopped buying butter and looked for meat with the fat trimmed off.

In 1977, when the first *Dietary Goals for the United States* document was released, the average American was eating just over 39 kilograms of beef a year. By 2008, that had dropped to just under 28 kilograms, a fall of almost 30 per cent. But chicken consumption more than doubled from 13 kilograms in 1977 to almost 27 kilograms in 2008, and turkey consumption shot from 3 to 6 kilograms in the same period.

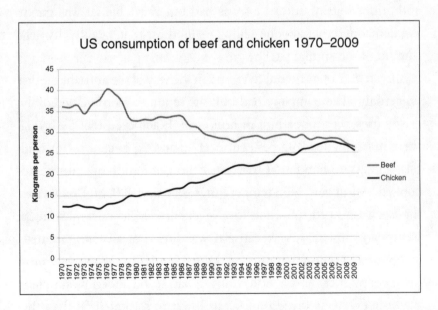

We don't eat as much turkey here, but Australian statistics are equally impressive. We listened hard when the government told us to eat less saturated fat, which it said was in red meat. We managed to more than halve our consumption of animal fat from 15 kilograms per person per year in 1969 to just 6 kilograms in 1999. And just like our American friends, our total meat consumption has increased only slightly, and we've changed the mix in favour of what we're told are lean meats.

While chicken farmers would certainly have been happy with the guidelines, the real winners were the makers of polyunsaturated vegetable and seed oils. For vegetable-oil manufacturers, the anti-animal-fat message was a gift from the marketing gods, and it was a gift they didn't intend to squander. People started buying margarine in preference to butter; vegetable oil rather than animal fat was used in the deep fryer because it was 'healthier'; and vegetable shortenings started being used in commercial baked foods from crackers to crisps. The polyunsaturated-oil industry exploded. The authorities told us animal fat was bad but vegetable fat was good. We demanded that anyone selling us food make it 'healthy' by getting rid of the animal fat.

Even McDonald's couldn't stand in the way of the anti-animal-fat juggernaut. The company had built its reputation on its incredibly crispy fries with just a hint of beef taste. It achieved that by frying them in beef tallow (93 per cent beef fat and 7 per cent cottonseed oil), an easy-to-handle fat that was solid at room temperature and cooked fries at very high temperatures. But by 1990, McDonald's in the US was forced to switch to a vegetable-oil blend. It was much more dangerous to use because it was liquid at all temperatures; it fried at a lower temperature, making it harder to consistently produce crispy fries; and beef flavouring had to be added to simulate the taste everyone loved. But it was lower in saturated fat than the tallow and McDonald's could therefore advertise it as a 'healthy' improvement.

In 2004 McDonald's Australia followed suit (clearly we're slow learners here). And in 2006, McDonald's Australia changed the vegetable oil to a canola–sunflower blend with even lower saturated-fat content so it could earn a 'tick' of approval from the Australian Heart Foundation. KFC was one of the last major Australian fast-food vendors to resist the change to seed oils, But in 2009, it announced that it had finally caved in to the Australian Government's demands and replaced the palm oil it was using for deep-frying with a blend of canola and sunflower oils.

But Keys's saturated-fat theory is not the primary reason we're eating much more polyunsaturated fat now than at any time in history. Keys just gave the food-processing industry a halo to wear while they continued to do what they'd already been doing for more than half a century. The trend started long before the 1980s, and had everything to do with money and nothing to do with health.

The story of margarine

Throughout most of human history, butter-making has required a close interaction between milkmaids, cows and butter churns. All that labour produced a very desirable product, but the price meant there was room for competition. In the middle of the 19th century, rapidly growing human populations meant demand for butter was pushing the price relentlessly higher. In 1869, the French emperor, Napoleon III, offered a prize to anyone who could develop a substitute for butter that could be used by the armed forces and the lower classes (there was no risk that he'd be eating the stuff, but the peasants could eat it if it was cheap).

A chemist by the name of Hippolyte Mège-Mouriès had the brilliant idea of applying a lard (pig-fat) modification process that had been used to make cheap oil lamps and candles to create an edible but cheap spread. The industrial revolution had significantly increased the demand for oils that could be used instead of beeswax or spermaceti (a wax from the head of the sperm whale) as lubricants and in lamps. French chemists had created a way of producing a usable oil (oleo oil) and a usable wax-like fat (oleostearine) from lard. By the late 1700s the French were making cheaper candles out of the oleostearine and putting cheap oleo oil in their lamps.

Mège-Mouriès figured out how to make a butter-like spread from a mixture of the oleo oil and the oleostearine. He called it oleomargarine and patented it immediately, but it seems the choosy French public was less than impressed, because the product bombed. Apparently, about the only thing it had going for it was that it didn't kill you. In 1871, Mège-Mouriès sold the patent and his operations to a Dutch company that ultimately became part of the multinational food conglomerate today called Unilever, the maker of Flora margarine in Australia, among very many other things.

The rapid urbanisation of North America in the 1870s meant that demand for a cheap substitute for butter and shortening (fats used to bake breads and other pastries) was intense. The margarine and shortening industries expanded quickly, using processes similar to those invented by Mège-Mouriès, but with an American twist. America had vast quantities of cottonseed oil, a useless by-product of cottonseed pressing (which produced the cottonseed linters used as stuffing for mattresses and upholstery, and cottonseed meal used for animal feed). In the US, margarine and shortening changed quickly from being based largely on pig fat to being based largely on cottonseed oil. The new cottonseed-oil products were marketed widely as a cheap substitute for lard (pig fat) and tallow (beef fat).

The problem was that cottonseed oil is liquid at room temperature, and the only way to make it solid was to mix it with animal fats produced from the processing of lard and tallow. It was a constant source of irritation for the processed-oil industries that they were dependent on their primary competitors – the slaughterhouses – for a key ingredient in their product.

Hydrogenation and Crisco

In 1901 the problem was solved with the invention of hydrogenation. If hydrogen was introduced to liquid vegetable oils under extreme heat, the polyunsaturated fatty acids would become partially saturated with hydrogen and produce nice straight fatty-acid molecules that solidified just like butter. The brand-new invention of hydrogenation allowed Procter & Gamble (previously a soap company) to introduce the first vegetable-based shortening, Crisco (for **cry**stallised **c**otton **oil**). Crisco was completely free of animal fat, and Procter & Gamble played that fact to the hilt in its advertising. The complete lack of moo-cows in the process meant Crisco could be sold considerably cheaper than lard, and the market just loved that.

Crisco

Procter & Gamble didn't invent hydrogenated oils. The process of 'fat hardening' was invented in 1901 by Wilhelm Normann, a German chemist working for a machine-oil factory. While trying to develop an inexpensive alternative to tallow (beef fat) for machine lubrication, he discovered that if he boiled cottonseed oil at 260°C in the presence of copper, he could produce a solid fat that looked and most importantly lubricated machines just like tallow.

He sold his patent in 1908 to a British soap manufacturer that saw potential in the hardened fat as a cheap way to make soap, which normally required tallow. The chemist in charge of the process was lured away from the British firm by the huge American soap manufacturer Procter & Gamble. The plan was to completely

---

153

harden the oils to make the raw materials for soap, but the temptation to sell the product as food was too great. It looked like lard and it cooked like lard, so why not sell it as cheap lard? By 1911, Crisco shortening was appearing on grocery-store shelves.

At the time, American housewives cooked with lard and butter. Procter & Gamble faced a huge marketing challenge in convincing them that the new product was better than those their mothers, grandmothers and great-grandmothers had used for centuries. Crisco was advertised as a healthier alternative to animal fats and more economical than butter. There was no justification to the health claim, it just sounded good in the ad copy.

Crisco lived up to the hype. It did cook just like lard and it was significantly cheaper. It became popular almost immediately. Sales volumes exploded from a mere 2.6 million pounds (1.2 million kilograms) in 1912 to 60 million pounds (27.2 million kilograms) just four years later.

The explosion in seed-oil use

By the start of World War I, hydrogenation was all the rage, and a good thing too, because butter and animal fat were about to be in short supply. Consumption of hydrogenated cottonseed oils in the form of margarines and shortenings expanded rapidly, and that drew many farmers into producing cottonseed, so much so that by 1933, laws were passed to reduce the surplus cottonseed acreages.

This presented an opportunity for another seed oil, soybean oil, which although it was even cheaper had until then been playing second fiddle to cottonseed. Its use skyrocketed in the 1930s and rose even more dramatically during World War II. By 1944, soybean oil accounted for 50 per cent of the fats used in shortening, up from 0.2 per cent just one decade earlier.

By 1967, seed-oil-based shortening accounted for almost a third of all fats consumed in the US; seed-based salad and cooking oils accounted for almost a further third; and seed-oil-based margarine made up almost a quarter. The remaining 14 per cent was animal-fat-based shortenings and butter. Just 60 years earlier, those numbers had been the complete opposite – 90 per cent animal-based.

Seed oil was well and truly on the rise at the expense of animal fat, but a huge boost for the seed-oil manufacturers was just around the corner. Ancel Keys was lobbying hard for the Mediterranean diet and telling us that the reason for the heart-disease epidemic was a significant increase in our consumption of animal fats.

The ironic reality was that, whether we knew it or not, by then we'd been steadily reducing our animal-fat consumption since the start of the century. If anything, the argument could have been that the increase in seed-oil consumption was to blame for the heart-disease epidemic, but if he knew those details, Keys didn't let them get in the way of the story he had to tell. The food processors realised their opportunity and swung in behind the Keys message with all the marketing power they could muster.

By 1967, about two-thirds of all seed-oil shortening was sold to potato-chippers, bakers, fast-food chains, other food manufacturers and restaurants. Institutional use also increased very rapidly. Since 1961, shortening had been produced with a higher content of polyunsaturated fatty acids – 22–35 per cent versus 6–15 per cent previously. The food industry preferred a higher polyunsaturated-fat content, because it made the oil flow more easily and made it easier to handle at room temperature. It preferred oils that flowed like olive oil rather than honey. And it very much preferred the price of soy-based shortenings to the price of lard. By 1968, liquid shortenings containing 30–50 per cent polyunsaturated fat were commonly being used in food processing and production, mostly because they were cheaper and easier to use. But thanks to Dr Keys and the American Heart Association, their use could be justified on the basis that they were healthy as well.

There aren't too many times in business when doing the cheapest thing coincides with doing the thing the health authorities want you to, but this was one of those times. The food processors must have (quietly) jumped for joy.

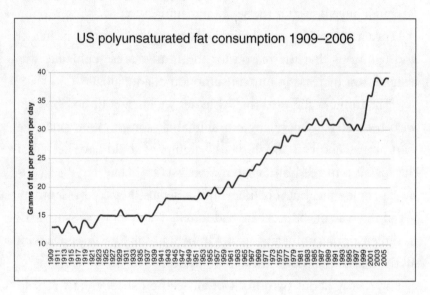

The health pronouncements of the 1970s and 1980s sealed (or perhaps just hurried) the fate of animal fats. By the 1980s, it became almost impossible to buy lard in a supermarket, and the primary consumers of animal-fat-based products are now pet-food and soap manufacturers.

Trans fats

In the 100 years from 1880 to 1980, seed-oil-based polyunsaturated fats completely replaced animal fats in the food-processing industry. But there was a grey cloud on the horizon. The process that permitted the massive expansion in the use of soybean oil was hydrogenation. Hydrogenation makes a thin vegetable oil thicker and even solid (depending on need) by turning polyunsaturated fats into molecules that look more like monounsaturated fats, which are nice and straight so pack together more easily (see Chapter 7). Unfortunately, the trans fats produced by the hydrogenation process are not exactly the same as the monounsaturated fats they imitate. In a true monounsaturated fat, the two carbon atoms linked by a double bond have hydrogen atoms attached to the same side of the fatty-acid chain – this is called a *cis* arrangement (see below left). But in a hydrogenated fat, the two double-bonded carbon atoms have the hydrogen atoms attached on opposite sides of the fatty-acid chain – this is called a *trans* arrangement (see below right).

$$\begin{array}{cc} \text{H} \quad \text{H} & \text{H} \\ \text{C} = \text{C} & \text{C} = \text{C} \\ & \text{H} \end{array}$$

A fatty acid with the trans arrangement, also known as a trans fat, works just the same as a normal fat in cooking, but during the early 1990s, evidence started to emerge that once these fats are inside our bodies, they significantly increase our risk of heart disease. They do this by decreasing HDL cholesterol – more on that coming up on page 167. A series of human studies in the UK produced consistent evidence that trans fats also significantly increase the chances of type 2 diabetes. And, much more worrying, studies on breastfeeding mothers who were eating diets high in hydrogenated seed oils showed that up to 17 per cent of the fats in their breast milk was trans fat (whereas it would normally be less than 1 per cent). The babies of those women had significantly lower visual-acuity scores than babies whose mother had not eaten trans fats.

Hydrogenated soybean oil was 25–50 per cent trans fat, so the 1990s research was a marketing crisis for the seed-oil industry.

The health message being spread by Dr Keys and the American Heart Association at the time was that saturated fats were bad, but polyunsaturated and monounsaturated fats were good. Soybean oil was largely polyunsaturated to begin with, but once it was hydrogenated it contained significant quantities of trans fats, which were not separately identified on food labels at the time.

The officially healthy oils, such as olive oil, are largely monounsaturated (see Chapter 7), which means they're thicker and don't need to be hydrogenated for most uses. Olive oil seemed the ideal alternative to the seed oils, but there was nowhere near enough of it, it would take a long time to establish new growers and its price was prohibitive anyway. If the food processors had to pay that much for their oil, they might as well be using animal fats. The obvious solution was to switch from soy-based oils to an oil that was much higher in monounsaturated fats but was also cheap. Canola oil fitted the bill perfectly.

Canola oil

Canola (from **Can**adian **o**il **l**ow **a**cid) was bred from rapeseed plants in the late 1970s. Introduced towards the end of the 1980s, it was a perfect substitute for olive oil (and in turn for soybean oil) because it was high in monounsaturated fats but (relative to soybean oil) low in saturated fats. In 1998, the first genetically engineered canola was introduced.

Oil	Saturated fat (%)	Monounsaturated fat (%)	Polyunsaturated fat (%)
Unhydrogenated soybean	18	24	58
Olive	17	74	9
Unhydrogenated canola	6	67	27

Because canola oil has fewer polyunsaturated fats than soybean oil, it didn't require as much hydrogenation and had about half the trans fats of soybean oil, which was still quite a bit. The widespread introduction of canola oil meant that polyunsaturated-fat consumption flattened in the 1990s, but the switch by most fast-food operators (such as McDonald's) away from lard-based frying to seed oils towards the end of the decade boosted consumption of polyunsaturated oils enormously.

Canola-oil use in the US has come from nothing in 2000 to about 20 per cent of all vegetable oils today. In Australia, canola represents about 45 per cent of oil consumed. From a minor crop in the late 1980s, canola is now Australia's third-largest broad-acre crop (after wheat and barley) and we now supply 20 per cent of the world market.

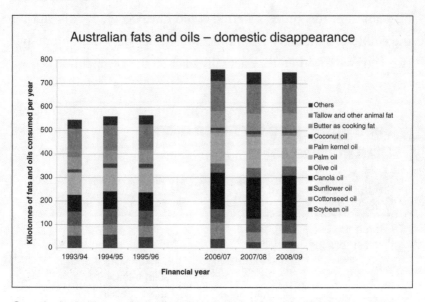

Over the last 15 years Australian consumption of canola oil has increased 2.4 times. Another major change has been that only around 50 per cent of the animal-fat consumption is now in the food industry, with the balance going to the chemical and the biofuels industries. (*Source*: Australian Oilseed Federation)

The seed-oil industry

The story of the seed-oil industry is the story of industrial food on a grand scale. It is the application of man's intelligence to the problem of demand versus supply. Edible seed oils were invented because a gap opened in the market. Animal fats could not supply the extreme urbanisation occurring on the American continent at anything like a reasonable price. Entrepreneurs discovered they could imitate the look, feel and utility of animal fats by using some smart chemistry and industrial processes.

Along the way, mistakes were made. Processes that looked innocent enough (such as hydrogenation) ended up causing more problems than they solved. But the enormous demand meant that the processed-food industry always had the resources to solve one technical problem with another. The explosion in heart disease 50 years after this process started could have been a PR disaster for the edible-oils industry, but miraculously, not only did no one put two and two together, they actually blamed the competition.

Seed oils – used for much more than margarine

Home use	The food-service industry	Food manufacturing

spreads
bottled oils for
  cooking
	spreads
	frying
	salad dressings
	cake and pastry
	  margarine
		pastry
		margarine, shortening
		liquid oils for frying
		solid fats for frying
		salad dressing oil
		spray oils
		dairy spreads
		coffee whiteners

The result is that now almost every fat we put in our mouth is a seed oil manufactured by an industry that didn't exist 100 years ago. And, even better – for the processors, at least – we're thanking them for saving us from dreaded animal fats, which sustained every generation of our human ancestors until the last two or three. But soy and canola farmers getting rich at the expense of cowboys is by far the least of our worries. The research now consistently shows that there's something very, very wrong with a diet where most of the fat comes from seed oils.

Modern biochemistry tells us that saturated fats and cholesterol are critical to the proper operation of the machine we walk around in. It also tells us that if we mess with the mix of fats we consume, we can significantly affect a cascade of important systems in our bodies. When we look at what the biochemistry actually says about how we process and use fats, the truth about dietary fats becomes abundantly clear. The advice we have been and continue to be given is not just wrong, it's seriously endangering our health.

9. POLYUNSATURATED FATS CAUSE HEART DISEASE – AND CHOLESTEROL DOESN'T

It's exceedingly difficult to find statistics on the number of people affected by heart disease over time. The official publications of the Australian Institute of Health and Welfare and the Australian Heart Foundation are full of glowing detail about the reduction in the number of deaths from cardiovascular diseases (heart disease, hypertension and stroke), from peaks in the late 1960s of about 60 000 (55 per cent of all deaths) a year. Nevertheless, cardiovascular disease (CVD) remains our biggest cause of death, killing 46 626 people (34 per cent of all deaths) in 2007.

Death rates have fallen because the medical profession has come to the rescue. We can detect heart disease earlier, manage it better and there are many more surgical options available as a last resort. But the bad news, which almost never makes it onto the front page, is that the prevalence of cardiovascular disease has dramatically increased. In the three decades from 1978 to 2008, the proportion of Australians living with CVD doubled, from 8 to 16.5 per cent. Many fewer people are dying as a result of heart disease, but it

162

does appear to be a 'Dutch boy with his finger in the dyke' effort on the part of the medical profession. Nothing has been done to slow the underlying cause of the disease, we've just got very good at making sure it kills fewer people – for now.

Throughout that time, the message from those who should know better has been that preventing heart disease is simple. All we need to do is reduce our saturated-fat and cholesterol intake. But it's been abundantly clear since the 1950s, and certain since the 1970s, that the amount of cholesterol and saturated fat we eat has absolutely nothing to do with our risk of heart disease. The American Heart Association and the Australian Heart Foundation drew a connection between dietary fat, cholesterol consumption and heart disease that the evidence just does not support. But much more recent research suggests that the oxidation of polyunsaturated fats transported with cholesterol in the bloodstream is likely to play a primary role in the development of heart disease.

What are plant sterols?

Only animals make cholesterol. Plants do, however, produce a class of chemicals very similar to cholesterol, called phytosterols or just plant sterols. Plant sterols are found in those plants and plant parts that are high in fat, such as seeds and nuts. Just like cholesterol in humans, plants use their sterols to provide flexibility in cell membranes and as the basis for a huge number of chemicals used in plant growth. Chemically there's almost no difference between a plant sterol and cholesterol.

An average Western diet has about as much plant sterol in it (200–400 milligrams per day) as it does cholesterol (200–500 milligrams per day). No one is quite sure why, but the presence of plant sterols in a food completely stops our intestine absorbing cholesterol, even though we absorb only about 1 per cent of the plant sterols we eat. The remarkable ability of plant sterols to stop cholesterol absorption was first noticed in 1951 and was immediately leapt upon by the drug companies. Eli Lilly brought out its first anti-cholesterol drug, Cytellin, in the late 1950s, but patients had to take 18 grams (4.5 teaspoons) of the stuff a day. That kind of quantity meant it was unmarketable as a drug and production quickly ceased.

The need to take such massive quantities of plant sterols before there was any observable effect on cholesterol levels kept them off the drug marketing agenda for three decades, helped along by the discovery of statins (see page 179). But by the early 1990s, a newly discovered method of combining plant sterols with fats dramatically decreased the amount needed to affect blood-cholesterol levels. A new industry was born and functional foods incorporating plant sterols started flooding onto the market. Initially they were just in margarines, but they quickly made their way into salad dressings, soy milks, yoghurts, cheeses, fruit drinks and even sausages and breads. In 2005, the then 10-year-old functional foods industry was already selling $3 billion worth of functional foods globally a year, including plant-sterol products, and growing rapidly.

More than 40 clinical studies on the effects of plant sterols have now been completed. There's absolutely no doubt that someone who regularly consumes plant sterols will reduce their blood-cholesterol levels by up to 6.8 per cent and their LDL cholesterol levels (see page 168) by up to 9.8 per cent. This means that plant sterols are very similar to statins (see page 179) in terms of their ability to reduce blood-cholesterol levels. But it's also clear that lowering blood-cholesterol levels doesn't improve heart-disease outcomes. Some recent studies have gone much further and even suggested that increased plant-sterol intakes are strongly associated with a significant increase in heart-disease risk.

One fact in no doubt at all is that plant sterols in the diet block the absorption of fat-soluble vitamins (particularly vitamin A), which is why people at risk of vitamin A deficiency should not consume foods containing added plant sterols.

The truth about cholesterol

Cholesterol is not a fat. It's a specialised form of alcohol produced by animals. Plants don't make it, but they do make an almost identical family of molecules called plant sterols (see page 163). Unlike most alcohols, cholesterol doesn't dissolve in water. Because of this handy little feature, animals like us weave it through our cell membranes to make our cells waterproof. Being waterproof is especially important around our electrical (nervous) system, so the greatest concentrations of cholesterol in our body are in the insulation (called myelin) around our nerves and in our brain. Our brain contains a quarter of all our cholesterol, even though it makes up only 2 per cent of our total weight.

Besides providing a waterproof structure for our cell membranes, which are made from fat (see Chapter 7), cholesterol is an essential precursor to many of our hormones. No cholesterol means no oestrogen and no testosterone, for example, which is why putting people on a low-fat diet is an extremely effective way to destroy their sexual desire.

Cholesterol is also critical in the formation of vitamin D by our body, and is a vital part of our own little damage-repair system. Scar tissue contains large amounts of cholesterol. And the older we get, it seems, the more critical the damage-repair system becomes. A 2011 study that followed 623 people aged 75 for an average of 17 years found that those with low blood cholesterol died 4.3 years earlier on average than folks with high blood cholesterol.

Our bodies make huge quantities of the stuff. Almost every cell in our body makes cholesterol, although the vast majority is manufactured in the liver. The average adult has 10 000 to 14 000 milligrams in circulation at any one time. We make as much as we need and automatically adjust the amount we make to take account of the amount we eat. This is why studies have repeatedly shown that feeding people cholesterol has a minimal effect on their blood-cholesterol readings.

We have a complex feedback system to make sure we don't make cholesterol if it's already in our food. Herbivores such as rabbits, however, don't have such a system – they don't need it, since their normal diet doesn't include cholesterol – which is why feeding cholesterol to rabbits pushed their blood-cholesterol readings through the roof (see Chapter 8).

But there's strong evidence that if we eat too little cholesterol, our bodies can't make quite enough to make up the difference, so it's important to ensure we get enough in our diet. Like all meat-eaters, we seem to have been built on the assumption that there'll be some cholesterol in our diet. The current dietary advice is to restrict our consumption of dietary cholesterol to less than 300 milligrams per day (an egg yolk alone contains 250 milligrams). Tossing 300 milligrams into a circulating pool of 14 000 milligrams would have almost no measurable effect, even if we weren't compensating anyway. But if we take that advice seriously, we can dramatically deplete our cholesterol levels over time.

Good, bad and ugly cholesterol

Contrary to popular belief there's only one kind of cholesterol. There's no good, bad (or even ugly) cholesterol. There's just cholesterol. It forms the structure that holds together and waterproofs our fat-walled cell membranes. It also forms the structure that holds together the globules of fat being transported in our bloodstream. We need to get the fat from our intestines to the cells that need it (see Chapter 7). Since our blood is a water-based solution and fat doesn't dissolve in water, this presents a bit of problem in the logistics department. That's where lipoproteins (*lipo* meaning 'fat') come in. If we didn't have lipoproteins, our blood would be like milk straight from the cow, with a layer of fat-based cream floating on a layer of water-based milk. Our body packages the fat and cholesterol with lipoproteins in a bundle of molecules ready for shipping. In the analogy I used in Chapter 7, the lipoproteins are the semi-trailers in our city-body, and the cholesterol is the shipping containers. Safe inside the shipping containers is the fat that needs to be transported around the body.

Semi-trailers and shipping containers are not a perfect analogy because, unlike a steel container, lipoproteins are very flexible and they reside on the inside of the load rather than the outside, but stick with me for a minute. If our little lipoprotein semi-trailers are loaded up with just the right amount of fat – and of course cholesterol to bind it all together – they're large and fluffy. So in reality they're more like the World War II trucks that ran on gas with a big balloon on the roof.

These fluffy fat transporters are called low-density (because they take up a lot of space for very little mass) lipoproteins, or LDL cholesterol for short. It would be less confusing simply to call them LFT for large fat transporters, but science seems to revel in the obscure.

A different group of fat trucks roams our superhighways looking for any cholesterol or fat that the cells have decided they don't need. These high-density lipoprotein (HDL cholesterol) trucks can be thought of as recyclable-garbage disposal units. Most of the cholesterol in the blood (60–80 per cent) is transported by LDL. The rest is carried by HDL. The HDL trucks cruise the system looking for any usable leftovers and take them back to the liver for repackaging on LDL trucks. Once again, a more helpful name for HDL cholesterol would have been FRT for fat-recycling transporters, but there you go.

Is HDL good and LDL bad?

LDL is often described as bad cholesterol and HDL as good cholesterol. This is because studies have shown that people with proportionally higher levels of HDL and lower levels of LDL in their blood are less prone to heart disease. That message has been pounded home by drug companies because the drugs used to lower cholesterol only affect LDL cholesterol.

When a doctor says you have a high 'bad cholesterol' reading, they're talking about your LDL cholesterol being outside a target range of 2.6–3.3 mmol/L. If you get too far out of that range – greater than 6.5 mmol/L – out will come the prescription book and there's a good chance you'll be prescribed drugs called statins (see page 179) to lower your LDL cholesterol levels.

If it's not quite that bad, your doctor may counsel you to lower your LDL cholesterol by eating more polyunsaturated fats. Both of these courses of action will lower LDL cholesterol but that won't necessarily affect your heart-disease risk.

LDL cholesterol and heart disease

People can be divided into two main groups according to whether their LDL cholesterol is large and fluffy or smaller and less fluffy. Some people have mostly large LDL particles and some people have mostly small ones. The folks with the large particles are are said to be Pattern A and those with smaller, less fluffy particles are Pattern B.

Pattern B LDL particles are deficient in cholesterol – they don't have enough structure for all the fat they're carrying. A low-fat, low-cholesterol diet is likely to push us into having more overloaded (or Pattern B) particles than will a high-fat, high-cholesterol diet. That theory has been repeatedly backed up by observations of people on extremely low-fat diets. One of the first examples was a study published in 1999 by a University of California, Berkeley research team. They found that if you put a Pattern A (large fluffy LDL) person on an extremely low-fat diet (that is, one in which less than 25 per cent of the total calories came from fat), they change to Pattern B (small dense LDL).

A much more recent study, completed in Queensland in 2010, backed up that observation and connected it to death from heart disease. The 16-year study followed the dairy consumption of 1529 Australians aged 25–78. The participants were asked about their dairy intake on three occasions (in 1992, 1994 and 1996). The results were then cross-matched to National Death Index data from 1992 to 2007. The data showed a significant relationship between the consumption of full-fat dairy and heart-disease deaths, but not the one you might think. The people who consumed full-fat dairy had a 69 per cent lower risk of death by heart attack than those gritting their teeth and gulping down low-fat milk. The people doing everything right – according to the guidelines – were most likely to end up dead from a heart attack.

If you wanted to convert someone from Pattern A (large fluffy LDL) to Pattern B (small dense LDL), you could restrict their dietary-cholesterol intake by putting them on a low-fat diet or you could put them on a high-fructose diet. Fructose is converted directly to fat by the liver, but because it's consumed as a sugar, it doesn't come with the accompanying cholesterol you'd normally get as part of a high-fat diet. The result is the overloaded fat trucks typical of Pattern B.

This theory was put to the test by a study published in 2007. The researchers measured the LDL particle size of groups of normal and overweight Swiss schoolchildren, and compared the results to the amount of fructose consumed. They found that the more fructose a child ate, the more likely they were to have Pattern B LDL particles.

Which cholesterol pattern you are matters, because if you're Pattern A, your LDL reading is *not* an indicator of heart-disease risk. But Pattern B people are at three times the heart-disease risk of Pattern A people. This is because Pattern A LDL particles are much less prone to oxidation. The more cholesterol an LDL particle has, the larger and more buoyant (fluffy) it is and the less likely it is to oxidise.

Are eggs really bad for you?

Eggs are almost perfect foods – they contain all the vitamins and minerals we require in the proportions we need them. But in the 1980s, eggs were demonised by the health authorities because the yolk has a high cholesterol content.

We were warned to moderate our consumption of eggs and particularly egg yolks, which kicked off a craze for egg-white omelettes. Most crustaceans (prawns, crabs, and so on) are similarly high in cholesterol, but for some reason they missed out on the vilification – perhaps they have a better marketing department.

From 1984 to 1988, US egg sales fell $1 billion to $3.1 billion, and the number of US egg producers was cut almost in half. But by 1999, studies were starting to suggest that, while eggs certainly do contain plenty of cholesterol, there's absolutely no association between egg consumption and our chances of heart disease. Two major trials involving more than 110 000 people found that we're no more likely to have heart disease if we eat more than an egg a day than if we eat less than an egg a week.

It's taken a while for that truth to percolate through to the Australian *Dietary Guidelines*, but tucked away in the fine print of the 2003 version is a recommendation to eat an egg a day to keep the doctor away. Strangely, the hypocrisy of recommending a very high-cholesterol food and simultaneously telling us to reduce our cholesterol has escaped the authors.

Perhaps one of the greatest previously unknown benefits of eggs was revealed in a 2006 review of the research on egg consumption. It concluded that eggs were an extremely effective way of converting a person from Pattern B to Pattern A (see 'LDL cholesterol and heart disease', on page 168). This is likely to be because eggs, being high in cholesterol, topped up the cholesterol levels available for making LDL particles, meaning the larger particles could once again be manufactured and the person became Pattern A again.

LDL cholesterol and oxidation

If the LDL particles are transporting large cargos of polyunsaturated fats, they can become the victims of out-of-control oxidation, the process that turns fat into rancid fat. Temperature affects the speed of oxidation, which is why oils that are largely made of polyunsaturated fats go rancid (or oxidise) so quickly at room temperature. Margarine left out of the fridge will go rancid much more quickly than butter because it contains a much higher proportion of polyunsaturated fats. The more double (unsaturated) bonds there are in a fat, the more rapidly it will oxidise or go rancid. When you store those fats at body temperature (which is 37°C, a good 15°C higher than average room temperature), they oxidise very quickly indeed.

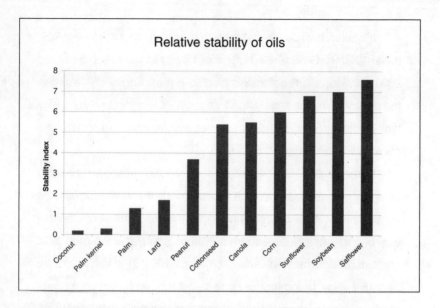

Relative stability of oils

Relative rate of oxygen reactivity for the common food oils. An oil with a stability index of 1 is highly stable. An index of 10 means it's highly unstable. (*Source*: Australian Oilseed Federation)

Oxygen reacts with the more reactive double carbon bonds found in unsaturated fats (see page 124). The reaction creates a class of chemicals called a lipid or fat radical, a type of free radical. Free radicals are extremely reactive and unstable molecules. Just like starting an uncontrolled fire, the free radicals start a chain reaction of oxidation in nearby polyunsaturates. Oxygen continues to react with other available unsaturated double bonds and the whole process results in many of the unsaturated fats being cut apart. This in turn causes significant damage to LDL particles and the release of some harmful classes of chemicals into the body. Our bodies didn't fall off the back of a truck yesterday, so we're well equipped with defences against out-of-control oxidation. We can normally use anti-oxidants to shut down that kind of chain reaction before it does any real damage – they're our own little fire suppressors.

Anti-oxidants in margarines

Anti-oxidants are often added to margarines to stop them going rancid so quickly. They'll often appear on the food label as a 'preservative' and have a number such as E320 (butylated hydroxyanisole – a popular choice). But sometimes they'll appear on the front of the label and be touted as a benefit – 'contains anti-oxidants' – depending on how much the food manufacturer thinks we know about anti-oxidants. They're not there to make you healthy but to stop your margarine going off.

Anti-oxidants are chemicals that stop or slow oxidation. Our bodies make anti-oxidants. If we have normal (pre-seed-oil) levels of unsaturated fats, our body can produce all the anti-oxidants it needs to combat any real oxidative damage. But our production systems are limited. If we pump up the amount of polyunsaturated fat in our system, we quickly run out of anti-oxidants and our bodies enter oxidative stress, which simply means that the balance between oxidation and anti-oxidation gets out of kilter. I like to think of it as an out-of-control bushfire (fire is actually just rapid oxidation – no oxygen, no fire).

LDL particles are carrying flammable cargo in a bloodstream full of oxygen, so the liver creates a supply of anti-oxidants (predominantly vitamin E and coenzyme Q10; I think of them as onboard fire extinguishers) when it loads them up for the trip. But the more polyunsaturated fats and the less cholesterol (which inhibits oxidation) in the load, the more likely the LDL particle is to run out of anti-oxidants before it gets to the cells that need its cargo.

If an LDL particle starts to oxidise (burn) out of control, it's described as oxidised LDL. But our bodies are ready for that eventuality as well. Certain types of immune cells called macro-phages have receptors for oxidised LDL particles. They keep an eye out on the highway for any oxidised LDL trucks careering out of control, then grab them and engulf them before they can do any damage. Once again, this all works well only if the amount of oxi-dised LDL is within our normal (pre-seed-oil) limits.

Oxidised LDL and heart disease

Oxidised LDL can be measured directly in blood tests and is an extremely accurate way of predicting heart disease. A 2001 study from the University of Belgium compared traditional predictors (such as total cholesterol, LDL levels and HDL levels) with a meas-ure of oxidised LDL. They found the traditional method was right only 20 per cent of the time (which means you'd do much better tossing a coin), but oxidised LDL levels predicted correctly 76 per cent of the time.

Those big fluffy LDL fat transporters are our body's way of trans-porting vital supplies to the cells that need energy and building materials. As long as the LDL can make it along the highway (our bloodstream) without being oxidised, it will accomplish that task perfectly. Older studies identified a limited association between LDL cholesterol levels and heart disease, but in fact those people at high risk probably also had much higher levels of oxidised LDL (which couldn't be measured when those studies were done). This is also likely to explain why some people can have a high LDL reading and no heart disease, while others can have a low LDL reading yet die from a heart attack. It isn't the gross LDL reading that matters, it's the percentage of *oxidised* LDL that's critical.

Many things affect the likelihood of oxidation. We know that HDL cholesterol (the fat-recycling trucks) have a much higher proportion of anti-oxidant cargo than LDL trucks. Since 1981, researchers have known that a great way to stop a solution of LDL oxidising is simply add some HDL. The higher anti-oxidant proportion puts out the fires (stops the oxidation). This mechanism very neatly explains why multiple trials have observed that a patient with high HDL (or 'good' cholesterol) is much less likely to be affected by heart disease than one with low HDL.

Fructose and oxidation of LDL

We also know that increasing the amount of fructose in the diet can dramatically increase oxidation of LDL. Besides shifting people to Pattern B (small dense LDL; see above), fructose decreases the production of nitric oxide, a powerful anti-oxidant, and significantly accelerates the creation of AGEs (see Chapter 6) and reactive oxygen species (fuel that keeps the oxidation fire burning). The association between sugar and heart disease was most recently confirmed in a major study published in 2010.

In that study, 6113 average American adults were divided into five groups based on their sugar consumption. One group was a standout on many of the traditional measures for heart-disease risk. They had the lowest fat consumption (just 28.9 per cent of total calories; the Australian Heart Foundation recommends keeping it under 35 per cent). They had the lowest saturated-fat consumption (just 9.7 per cent of total calories). And they had the lowest cholesterol intake by a country mile (only 238 milligrams per day).

This group were poster children for the low-fat lifestyle. There was just one little problem: their blood work was awful. On average, the folks in the low-fat group had by far the worst blood-cholesterol and triglyceride (the amount of fat in the blood; see page 127) readings of all five groups studied. And they weren't just bad, they were 'time to order some drugs' bad. The people doing everything right from a fat-consumption perspective were most likely to end up dead from a heart attack. They were also eating the most sugar.

Combining a high-sugar (high-fructose) diet with a high intake of polyunsaturated fat appears to create the perfect environment for oxidised LDL – in fact, I think we'd really be hard pressed to invent a better environment. And the research now clearly shows that the oxidation of LDL cholesterol (rather than the mere consumption of dietary cholesterol) is a primary cause of heart disease.

LDL and the formation of atherosclerotic lesions

Once our LDL transports are set on fire (oxidised) they become dangerous mutants. They're packed with the burned half-remains of unsaturated fats and they're small and heavy. Our cells no longer recognise them as useful, our liver doesn't recycle them and they continue to circulate in our bloodstream. Most get slurped up by our ever-vigilant defenders in the immune system, but when there are just too many (such as when we eat lots of polyunsaturated fats), some end up embedded in the cells lining our arterial walls. This is made all the easier by fructose consumption: nitric oxide is essential for keeping the arterial linings impervious to LDL penetration, and fructose depresses the production of nitric oxide.

How LDL gets across the arterial walls

The interior lining of our arteries is called the endothelium (from the Latin *endo*, 'inside', and the Greek *thele*, 'nipple' – go figure). Endothelial cells are packed very closely together to form a sheet, but there are narrow gaps between them that allow small particles to pass back and forth through the artery wall. These gaps, which are around 26 nanometres in diameter (about the same size as a particle of wood smoke), give the artery vital access to the oxygen and other chemicals in the blood.

The smaller an LDL particle, the more likely it is to be able to cross the wall through one of these gaps. Pattern A LDL particles are just a little bit too big (26.3–30 nanometres) to get through the gaps between the endothelial cells and so cannot get stuck in the arterial wall. Pattern B LDL particles (which are just 5 per cent smaller on average) are taken up by the arterial wall at a 50 per cent greater rate. LDL particles that are less than 25.8 nanometres in diameter can get through the holes easily, and that's where the problems start.

Once the LDL particle is embedded in the arterial wall, its load of oxidised rubbish is deposited in the cells lining the arteries. Our immune system immediately recognises that rubbish as something that needs to be disposed of and attacks it. This would normally be a good idea, except now these molecules are embedded in our arterial walls, so our immune system attacks our own arteries.

This is why the atherosclerotic lesions (see page 133) in our arterial walls are always filled with dead immune cells and loads of oxidised LDL. Our highway clearance system does its best with the wreckage that crashes into the artery walls, but when we have too much oxidised LDL, the immune-system macrophages become part of the problem rather than the solution. We end up with lesions filled with oxidised LDL and with the foam cells that our macrophages become when they ingest that LDL.

If I were of a nasty disposition and wanted to recommend a diet that was sure to give you heart disease, there could be no better way than tell you to avoid animal fat and make sure you consume lots

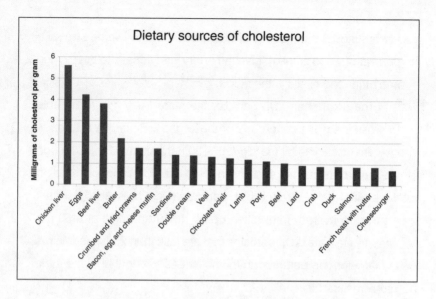

of polyunsaturated seed oils (which have no cholesterol). That way your poor little LDL transports would be overloaded with highly flammable polyunsaturated cargo and you wouldn't have enough cholesterol to make them a decent size. You'd be dead from heart disease in no time flat. The only problem is that the diet I've just suggested is exactly the diet being recommended to us every day by the *Dietary Guidelines for Australians*. Now that's a bit of a problem.

Are drugs the answer?

The folks squeezing oil out of soybeans and canola seeds are not the only people making money out of the 'cholesterol gives you heart disease' story. In keeping with the theme that there's no money in telling people NOT to eat something, the solution we've been offered for the perceived problem of high cholesterol is to take drugs. The pharmaceutical industry saw the market potential early and immediately set out to find drugs that would lower our choles-terol readings.

Cholesterol is made when the liver uses an enzyme called HMG-CoA reductase to convert 7-dehydrocholesterol (don't worry, you don't need to remember that, although you might remember from Chapter 4 that we also use 7-dehydrocholesterol to create vitamin D). The target of drug-company research was to come up with something that stopped that enzyme working. The reasoning was simple: no enzyme means no cholesterol production and voilà – lower blood-cholesterol levels. The drug companies never bought for a minute the link between dietary cholesterol and blood cholesterol. All their efforts were targeted exclusively at shutting down the major source of cholesterol, our own liver.

The creation and marketing of statin drugs

In 1976, a Japanese researcher by the name of Akira Endo managed to isolate (from a citrus penicillin mould) a substance he called mevastatin that inhibited the action of HMG-CoA reductase. Word of Endo's discovery spread quickly, and by 1978 Merck & Co., one of the largest pharmaceutical companies in the world, was able to isolate a similar substance, which it called lovastatin. By 1987, Merck hit the market with Mevacor, the very first commercially available statin drug, based on lovastatin.

Before Mevacor, the only thing a doctor who followed the American Heart Association line could do for a patient with high blood cholesterol was suggest they eat less animal fat and more vegetable oils. Some early drugs had been tested before this time, but by 1987 the evidence was mounting that, while the drugs did lower LDL cholesterol, they didn't have any real effect on heart-disease outcomes.

The real problem for Merck, however, was not the competition, but that public awareness of the supposed link between cholesterol and heart disease was then pretty low. And if patients weren't worried, then neither were their doctors. Merck threw its considerable financial muscle into an 'education program', to ensure that the American public and their doctors became fully aware of just how dangerous cholesterol really was. The food industry saw its chance and piggybacked the campaign by marketing cholesterol-free foods. That publicity then fed back into the US Government's own publicity developed around the need to lower cholesterol (through eating fewer eggs and less animal fat), and the anti-cholesterol hysteria of the late 1980s and early 1990s was created.

Other drug companies started jumping on the bandwagon, and before long a new market segment in statin drugs had developed. The approval trials had shown the drugs did lower cholesterol (much more than and without all the nasty side effects of the first generation of drugs), but what was needed were trials that showed they actually changed heart-disease outcomes. In 1994, the 4S (Scandinavian Simvastatin Survival Study) trial came through with the goods. It had tested a new Merck statin – called simvastatin and later branded Zocor – on 4444 patients with high cholesterol who'd also already experienced heart attacks. After five years of simvastatin use, the average patient's LDL cholesterol fell by 35 per cent. But much more importantly, simvastatin had reduced the likelihood that a patient would die of a heart attack from 8.5 to 5 per cent (the drug company reported this as a 42 per cent improvement, which sounds much more impressive). Merck went to market with Zocor and by as early as 1995, it and Mevacor were each turning over $1 billion a year in sales for the company.

The honey pot was too big to ignore. In 1996, Pfizer (Merck's primary competitor) entered into an agreement with another company, Warner-Lambert, which had been struggling to get its statin called Lipitor ready for sale. Lipitor worked at lower doses than any of the competitors and lowered LDL cholesterol more (by 38 per cent). In 1997 Lipitor was ready for sale and drug reps went to work. Because of its lower dose, doctors thought it was safer and its price was also lower than most of the competition.

By June 1998, Lipitor had half the market share of Merck's drugs and was climbing fast. In 1999, Pfizer bought out Warner-Lambert for $90 billion. The drug companies lobbied hard for changes to the US guidelines on who should be prescribed cholesterol-lowering drugs, and in 2001 the guidelines were dramatically altered to recommend much more aggressive treatment of high cholesterol. This tripled the potential market for statins. By then – and in anticipation of the imminent release of AstraZeneca's Crestor – Pfizer decided to push Lipitor even harder, marketing it directly to consumers by saying: 'You don't have to be visibly unhealthy to have dangerously high cholesterol.'

The marketing paid off. By 2009, 25 per cent of Pfizer's profits were coming from Lipitor, and the worldwide market for all statins was estimated to be well over $25 billion per annum. In Australia, statins now chew up 13 per cent of the money paid out by the Pharmaceutical Benefits Scheme (PBS), and the amount shelled out for them by the Australian taxpayer (via the PBS) grew by 33 per cent in just the last year. The rest of the PBS combined grew by less than 5 per cent in the same period.

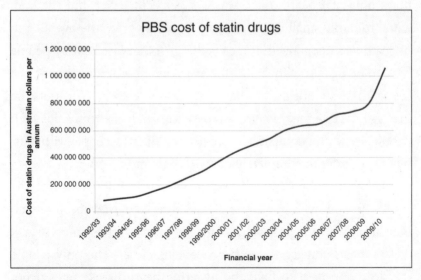

The cost to the Australian taxpayer of statin drugs – do you see a trend?

The case for and against statins

Statins do work. The 4S study showed that they do lower LDL cholesterol and they do reduce the chance of a heart-disease death in people who've already had a heart attack. But there's a good deal of evidence to suggest that the heart-disease improvements for these folks had nothing to do with the cholesterol-lowering and a lot to do with the interaction between the drug and other systems (such as blood-thinning). But 'people who've already suffered a heart attack' (and lived to tell the tale) is a very small market. The only way statin use could grow as rapidly as it has was to convince doctors to prescribe it and patients and the PBS to fund it for primary prevention among otherwise healthy people who've only been diagnosed with a higher than normal blood-cholesterol reading.

A comprehensive review published in 2007 of all of the major high-quality trials on statins concluded that for people in this primary-prevention category (who make up the overwhelming majority of those taking statins now) taking statins did not alter the overall risk of dying at all. The risk of statin-poppers suffering a non-fatal heart attack was 1.5 per cent lower, but that's an extraordinarily small improvement, especially given the overall risk of death was unchanged. It means that 67 otherwise healthy people have to be treated with statins for five years in order to prevent just one of them suffering a non-fatal heart-disease event. This puts the drugs in the category of being almost completely ineffective for such people. By way of comparison, we need to treat 11 people with antibiotics in order to completely cure 10 of them.

When the data were broken down by gender and age, the results became even less impressive. Statins conferred absolutely no benefit on women at all. And men aged over 69 (those most at risk of fatal heart attacks) enjoyed no benefits either. The only people the drug appeared to help (by lowering heart-disease rates if not death rates) were men aged 30–69, and then only by a very small absolute margin.

The reason for the disappointing results may be that the enzyme used to manufacture cholesterol, the one shut down by statin drugs, is also used to manufacture one of the primary anti-oxidants loaded onto the LDL trucks by the liver, co-enzyme Q10. Shutting down cholesterol production also means shutting down Q10 production. This might explain why, although these drugs have an enormous effect on cholesterol levels, they have a very limited effect on heart-disease outcomes. It might also be the case that although statins lower cholesterol, this has nothing to do with why they lower risks for people who've already had a heart attack. Just like aspirin, statins reduce clotting. And just like aspirin, statins provide the greatest benefit for those people who've already suffered a heart attack. But no one is ever going to make their fortune selling aspirin at 97 cents a box.

A series of studies has suggested relationships between statin usage, cancer, increased diabetes and cognitive impairment (memory loss in particular). But a significant independent review of the evidence of all trials, conducted in 2011 by the reliable Cochrane Review, found no significant evidence of statins causing cancer. It did, however, suggest that more investigation was needed into whether statins increase the incidence of type 2 diabetes and result in cognitive impairment and memory loss. The review also noted that the trials were almost all funded by drug companies and that there was significant evidence for selective reporting of results. It also noted that none of the trials had run for an extended term and there was no evidence that the drugs were safe to use for periods greater than 10 years. The review concluded by advising doctors to be cautious in prescribing statins to people who hadn't already had a heart attack.

Statins may be harmless, but some of the trials have raised real concerns about cognitive impairment and type 2 diabetes, and the jury is still well and truly out. Statins are powerful drugs that alter the function of important liver enzymes, and the evidence suggests that the only class of people that benefits from them significantly is younger men who've already had a heart attack, a rather small group. But this hasn't stopped the makers of statins lobbying for widespread preventative use and creating a multibillion-dollar industry that both feeds on and benefits from the myth that cholesterol has something to do with heart disease.

10. POLYUNSATURATED FATS CAUSE CANCER

Trials conducted in the 1960s and 1970s often lowered blood cholesterol by restricting the subjects' saturated-fat intake. They usually did this by replacing animal fats such as butter and lard with polyunsaturated fats such as corn oil, in the form of shortening, cooking oil and margarine.

One of the earliest of these human trials was the London Hospital Study, completed in 1965. In that study, 80 middle-aged men were randomly divided into three groups: one group was told to continue eating the normal British diet (you know the type of thing – fish and chips, black pudding and lamb's fry with a garnish of baked beans). Another group was told to replace animal fats with corn oil (60 per cent polyunsaturated fat). The last group replaced animal fats with olive oil (9 per cent polyunsaturated fat).

After two years, the corn-oil group had a blood-cholesterol level 25 per cent lower than that of the other two groups, which was perceived as very good news. But the bad news – and it was *very* bad news – was that 48 per cent of the corn-oil group and

43 per cent of the olive-oil group had suffered heart attacks in the meantime, while just 28 per cent of the full-fat group had suffered the same fate. The trial was dismissed at the time as being too small to raise concerns, but the researchers clearly stated that there was no evidence that feeding people polyunsaturated fat was likely to prevent heart disease.

A much larger trial, completed in 1971, was conducted with a population of 846 Californian military veterans randomly assigned to two different kitchens. In the Veterans Trial, one kitchen replaced all animal-fat products with corn oil for the eight-year duration of the study. The other kitchen kept on serving a normal high-animal-fat diet.

As expected, the corn-oil group had a lower average blood-cholesterol level, although the improvement (13 per cent) wasn't as great as in the London Hospital Study. Heart-disease-related events were slightly less than expected in both groups, but not significantly different from each other. But what really concerned the research-ers was the dramatic difference in cancer deaths between the two groups. The incidence of fatal cancers in the corn-oil group was nearly double that of the normal-diet group by the end of the eight-year trial.

The Veterans Trial was the last to replace animal fat with corn oil, and by far the largest and longest trial of its kind. It would be nice to have longer and relatively bigger trials like this, but they'd be unlikely to gain ethical approval (ethicists are so picky about doing things to people when you're testing the theory that your intervention will cause more cancer).

The good news is that Israel has been conducting its own unin-tentional trial of mass feeding with high doses of polyunsaturated fats for some time now. The Jewish population of Israel has taken to polyunsaturates like ducks to water. This is likely to be due to the requirement that food be kosher, which places significant restrictions on animal foods but not on vegetable foods. They have the world's highest concentration of polyunsaturated fats in their diet. In 1996, about 12 per cent of the energy they consumed came from polyunsaturated fats, compared to about 5 per cent in Australia at the same time.

But they also have some of the highest rates of heart disease, type 2 diabetes and most cancers. This is despite eating what could only be described as the perfect diet – high in polyunsaturated vegetable fats – according to our nutrition authorities. Often referred to in scientific journals as the 'Israeli paradox', this is the flip side of the 'French paradox' (the French have very low rates of these diseases and consume a diet very high in saturated fats). For non-Jewish Israelis, whose diet isn't high in polyunsaturated fats, the rate of diabetes is 1.5 times lower, of heart-disease deaths 2.3 times lower and of cancer 3.4 times lower. If you want to know what health statistics look like when you really follow the Australian Heart Foundation's advice, you need look no further than Israel.

Animal studies have been no more encouraging. Rat studies performed in the 1970s and 1980s consistently noted that mammary (breast) cancer was formed more often in rats fed corn oil (high in polyunsaturated fats) than in those fed coconut oil (high in saturated fats). And a truly disturbing study published in 1997 showed that feeding the rat equivalent of a breastfeeding mother a diet high in polyunsaturated fat (43 per cent corn oil) doubled the rate of mammary cancer in her daughters, caused cancers to appear among them earlier and caused earlier onset of puberty.

In 1996, Swedish researchers decided it was time for a human study to provide some hard data. Scientists from the Karolinska Institute recruited 63 870 women aged 40–76 and monitored their diet and the occurrence of breast cancer for an average of 4.2 years.

The dietary questionnaires used in the study enabled the researchers to determine exactly how much saturated, monounsaturated and polyunsaturated fat the women were consuming.

They found no association between the total fat or saturated-fat intake and a woman's risk of developing breast cancer. Consumption of monounsaturated fat reduced the risk of breast cancer by 20 per cent but polyunsaturated-fat consumption did the opposite. Just as the rat studies had predicted, the women consuming the most polyunsaturated fat were 20 per cent more likely to develop breast cancer than the women consuming the least.

Melanoma

Melanoma rates are the fastest growing of any cancer worldwide. Because it's the most easily diagnosed cancer, it's also the one for which we have the most reliable historic data. The official explanation is that melanoma is due to sun exposure, but the statistics make a mockery of that suggestion. Melanoma rates are not always highest in places with lots of sun. You're 10 times more likely to develop melanoma if you live in the Shetland Islands (north of Scotland) than if you live in the sunny Mediterranean. In Scotland there are five times as many cases of melanoma on the feet, which would almost never be exposed to sunlight, than on the hands, and in Japan 40 per cent of melanomas occur on the soles of the feet. Large recent studies of people who work outdoors have failed to find any significant association between the amount of time spent in the sun and the risk of melanoma.

That being said, rates of melanoma are extremely low among people with darker skin, and the darker the skin, the less melanoma there is. The presence or absence of melanin, the chemical that provides skin colouring, clearly has something to do with whether or not melanoma develops. But some very limited trials indicate that polyunsaturated fats may be a much more significant factor in the rapid increase of melanoma over the last 70 years.

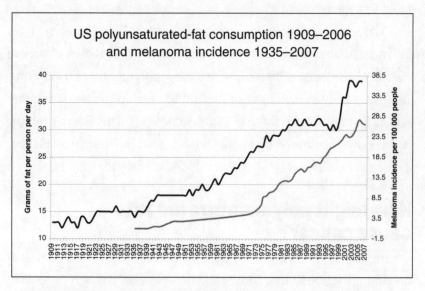

US polyunsaturated-fat consumption 1909–2006 and melanoma incidence 1935–2007

In Australia the equivalent rates are significantly higher. In 2000, the incidence of melanoma among Australian men was more than twice the US rate (53.7 per 100 000). The incidence of melanoma has accelerated in lockstep with polyunsaturated-fat consumption for the last 70 years. Is it really sensible to suggest the average American is getting 25 times as much sun now as they were in 1933?

Polyunsaturated fats and melanoma

In 1974, Dr Bruce Mackie noticed an unusual number of melanomas occurring among patients visiting his Sydney clinic (five patients in 12 weeks). He did a bit of digging and discovered that all five patients had, within the previous 10 months, replaced the animal fats in their diet with seed oils. Dr Mackie theorised that the melanomas were related to this dietary change. It took him a decade to arrange it, but eventually he put together a study with 100 melanoma patients and 100 controls without melanomas. He found that the melanoma patients all had significantly higher levels of polyunsaturated fats in their body fat just below the surface of their skin, while the controls had much lower levels of polyunsaturated fats there.

The study suggested a strong causative link between high polyunsaturated-fat consumption and cancer, and there's clearly a statistical association between increased polyunsaturated-fat consumption and the incidence of melanoma (just from comparing the rise in incidence with the rise in consumption). This doesn't tell us how a polyunsaturated fat might cause cancer, but there may just be a clue in the early work of doctors doing kidney transplants.

How might polyunsaturated fats cause cancer?

During the 1970s, UK kidney transplant surgeons theorised, based on animal studies, that since polyunsaturated fats suppress the immune system, they might be useful in stopping a transplant recipient's body attacking the transplant. They organised some trials using sunflower-seed oil, which is 68 per cent polyunsaturated. As predicted, the patients given the oil did much better than those left to their own devices. The seed oil suppressed the immune system and stopped it rejecting the transplant, but at about this time the results of the Veterans Trial (see page 186) raised concerns about large doses of polyunsaturated oils and increased cancer rates, so the practice was discontinued almost as soon as it was started.

The more unsaturated a fat is, the more bent its molecules are, because each unsaturated double bond (see Chapter 7) causes a kink in the carbon chain that makes up the fatty acid. This is why oils that contain a significant percentage of unsaturated fats (such as canola oil) are generally liquid at room temperature – they don't pack together that well. This, of course, means they're not a great choice for building cell membranes. It would be like trying to clad a house using any old branches you happened to find lying around. That kind of house might need quite a bit of extra structural framework to ensure the cladding stayed up.

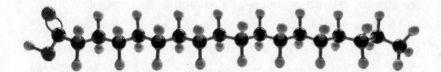

Stearic acid, a nice straight 18-carbon saturated fatty acid found in meat.

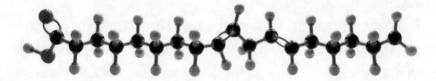

Linoleic acid – an 18-carbon polyunsaturated fat found in most seed oils – has two kinks at the unsaturated double bonds in the middle.

This is exactly what happens in our body. When we replace the saturated fats in our diet with unsaturated fats, our body just uses what we give it. It needs an 18-carbon fatty acid for cell membranes. If there are no saturated or monounsaturated 18-carbon fatty acids available, it will use an 18-carbon polyunsaturated fatty acid instead. That makes the cell membrane quite a bit limper than it would have been, so it uses extra cholesterol to stiffen things up a bit. This is why animal and human studies have shown time and time again that replacing saturated fat with polyunsaturated fat will lower the amount of cholesterol circulating in the bloodstream. Our little cell-builders are using more of it to shore up the dodgy work they've been doing with substandard building materials.

Because our bodies just use the fat we give them, a very direct way to measure how much polyunsaturated fat a person has been eating is to measure how much polyunsaturated fat is sitting in their fat tissues. The Jewish folk in Israel who'd been setting all kinds of records for polyunsaturated-fat consumption (see page 186) also had polyunsaturated-fat levels in their body fat that were off the scale – 25 per cent of the fat in their fat tissues was polyunsaturated. The normal (pre-20th-century) level should be less than 4 per cent. And Dr Mackie observed the same thing in his melanoma patients. Those with the melanomas had a lot more polyunsaturated fat in the cells just below the surface of the skin.

Polyunsaturated fats and oxidative stress

Having a bunch of polyunsaturated fats where the saturated fats should be doesn't just make for dodgy building work, it can also cause very direct harm. Polyunsaturates are more prone to uncontrolled oxidation at the points where they have the double carbon bonds (see Chapter 7).

Just like well-constructed Pattern A LDL particles (see page 168), a well-built cell membrane stuffed with saturated fats is very unlikely to suffer oxidative damage because it has few double carbon bonds for oxygen to attack. Building a cell membrane out of saturated and monounsaturated fats is like building the wall of a fireplace out of non-flammable bricks. But a cell membrane dominated by polyunsaturated fats is a different story: that's like building our fireplace out of balsa wood.

Out-of-control oxidation causes significant damage to the cell membrane and rampant production of free radicals. These free radicals (also called reactive oxygen species) can damage everything to do with a cell, from its membrane all the way down to the DNA. Oxidative damage has been clearly associated with heart disease and stroke, and it's easy to see why – if we're in oxidative stress, our insides are going rancid. Large-scale oxidation will result in oxidised LDL irreversibly damaging the arterial walls (see page 171). But it's the oxidative damage to our DNA that's likely to be the link between cancers and polyunsaturated seed oils.

DNA damage and cancer

Our cells normally die and replicate according to a schedule. They have DNA switches that tell them when they should replicate and when to die. If those DNA switches are damaged by oxidation on a massive scale, then the damaged cells can become a breeding ground for potential cancer growth. Cancer is the uncontrolled replication of cells. But cancer is not a single disease, it's hundreds (and probably thousands) of diseases. The reason cancer is treated as if it were a single disease is that cancers share many common characteristics.

Cancerous cells don't respond to the normal genetic signals telling them to stop growing, and their programmed cell death doesn't function as it should. They can persuade the surrounding tissue to provide them with a blood supply, they can trick our immune system into not seeing them as a threat, and they can invade our blood or lymphatic system and travel to other places in the body. Even the way each cancer cell achieves these magical feats of evasion and destruction is different from cell to cell. It takes billions of random, chaotic collapses of oxidised cells to produce cells with all of these characteristics. Our bodies need to be exposed to oxidation over very long time frames, but if they are, they will eventually produce the mutations that are lumped together under the general heading 'cancer'.

A study published in early 2011 looked in detail at the DNA of cancer cells, and it could only be described as a mess. It's like someone threw a grenade into the nucleus of a normal cell. Parts of the chromosomes (the strings of genes that decide what we are) have been chopped up and rearranged over and over – an average of 90 times in a prostate cancer tumour cell, for example. Even within tumours from the same cell type, there are huge variations in how the DNA has been rearranged.

Within any tumour, populations of cancer cells will be broken in very different ways. And as the tumour grows, this variation just increases. Finding a drug that has the same effect on all of these differently broken cells is the ongoing challenge for the cancer-treatment industry.

To stop this kind of damage occurring, our bodies come equipped with the ability to manufacture anti-oxidants. Like a fire on a freezing winter night, oxygen is paradoxically what we need to survive, but also extremely dangerous if we allow it to get out of control. We can control oxidation as long as we don't build our fire-places out of firewood. Unfortunately, the systems we use to control oxidation are built on the assumption that we won't be consuming vast amounts of polyunsaturated fats. And it's a valid assumption. We can't make polyunsaturated fats ourselves, and before the intro-duction of seed oils into our diet we were extremely unlikely to encounter them in any kind of quantity in our food. Before the processed-food industry figured out how to crush seeds at high temperatures and pressures to extract their polyunsaturated oils, no more than 5 per cent of the fat in our diet (and probably consider-ably less than that) was polyunsaturated fat, which came largely from fish and nuts.

Anything that causes cell damage can trigger a chain reaction of oxidation that can lead to oxidative stress and, if the right muta-tion occurs, cancer. And this might be the link between skin colour and melanoma. Melanin protects us from UVB radiation, which can penetrate the skin and damage the fat stored just below the surface. This mechanism is exactly the one we rely on to break down cholesterol and produce vitamin D (see Chapter 4). The UVB would usually also damage normal cell membranes, but because there'd be very few polyunsaturated fats present, any anti-oxidants could deal with it. If, however, those cell membranes were overloaded with polyunsaturated fats, their defences could be easily overcome, and oxidative stress and cancer could be the ultimate result.

Do anti-oxidant supplements work?

Drug companies, as always, have an answer – just top up your anti-oxidant supply. But trials of anti-oxidant supplements have been disappointing, to say the least. Vitamin E and beta-carotene, a plant precursor to vitamin A found in yellow–orange fruits such as cantaloupe (rockmelon) and vegetables such as carrots and green leafy vegetables, both occur naturally in vegetable oils to stop them going rancid as quickly as they otherwise might. Both are known to be powerful anti-oxidants, so they've been obvious candidates for trials of their ability to suppress cancer-causing oxidation.

In 1994, a major trial of the effectiveness of beta-carotene and vitamin E in cancer prevention was published. The researchers provided high-dose supplements to 29 000 smokers divided into three randomised groups taking beta-carotene, vitamin E or a placebo. After eight years, the researchers reported some truly worrying outcomes. The vitamin E group suffered significantly more strokes but their heart-disease and cancer outcomes were the same as those of the placebo group. Worse still, the beta-carotene group had much higher numbers of deaths from lung cancer and heart disease. Not only had the anti-oxidant supplements failed to prevent cancer, it looked like they'd made things worse. A trial of 18 000 people published two years later came to a similar conclusion about a supplement combining beta-carotene and vitamin A (also an anti-oxidant, found in meat and other animal products).

We don't know why supplementing with those anti-oxidants is more dangerous than not supplementing, but it might have something to do with the complexity of our oxidation-fighting equipment. The array of anti-oxidants produced by the body is huge, and the variety is not likely to be an accident. Perhaps if we detect vitamin E in our diet, we stop making our own. Perhaps changing the ratios of given anti-oxidants (such as vitamin A, vitamin E and beta-carotene) pushes something else out of balance and does more harm than good. But the real question is, why take the risk? The source of the oxidation problem in cell membranes is having too many poly-unsaturated fats in our diet. The cure is obvious and simple – don't eat polyunsaturated fats.

But there I go again, telling people NOT to do something. How does anybody make any money out of advice like that? The answer is they don't. The race is on in the commercial world to find anti-oxidant supplements that actually work. But if you don't want to wait that long and you want to make changes right now by cutting polyunsaturated fats and sugars out of your diet, then read on and I'll show you how.

PART 3

A PRACTICAL GUIDE TO AVOIDING SUGAR AND POLYUNSATURATED FATS

Introduction

If you've got this far in the book, you'll already know that diets requiring willpower (which is, ah, all of them) are pointless. That exercising to lose weight is possibly even more pointless. That the only thing gobbling vitamins will change is your bank balance. That you should get plenty of sunshine. And that there are much higher priorities for our diet than cutting down on salt.

You'll also have discovered that just two substances are making us fat and very, very sick – the fructose half of sugar and polyunsaturated seed oils. Neither of these substances was a material part of our diet before 1800, and even as recently as the 1930s, neither was eaten at lethal levels. But since then, our consumption of both has accelerated enormously, driven by two very simple principles – profit and cost. Sugar is addictive. If a food manufacturer adds it to their food they'll sell more. Seed oil is cheap. If a food manufacturer adds it to their food, that food will be cheaper to make. At no point in the history of the use of either of these substances has your health been a consideration, let alone a priority. If the substance doesn't

kill you on the spot, then it's all good as far as the food manufacturers are concerned, which explains the lack of hemlock in our
food supply.

If sugar or seed oils had not yet been invented, neither would
pass the testing required of a foodstuff today. Significant studies
show that much more testing, at the very least, is required before
sugar and seed oils could be certified as safe. If I invented gillespie-
ose oil today and attempted to have it accepted with the same kind
of research track record as either fructose or seed oil, I'd fail dismally.
The problem for us is that both substances were introduced into our
food supply just before regulators started controlling what was safe
to eat. By the time the regulators were invented, sugar and seed oils
were already 'generally regarded as safe', based on no greater fact
than nobody seemed to keel over after consuming them.

Neither sugar nor seed oils will kill you on the spot. And they
won't kill you the day after that or even a year later. Both substances
are slow-acting poisons that take decades to take effect. The research
clearly shows that taking both in serious quantities will result in
exactly the combination of chronic diseases that now afflict Australian society and are growing out of control. Fructose consumption
will make us fat, give us type 2 diabetes, fatty liver disease and
chronic kidney disease and, with help from seed oils, encourage
heart disease. Seed oils, apart from finishing the job on heart disease, will give us cancer.

There's no good (well, any) reason to consume sugar or polyunsaturated seed oils. They add not one single benefit and they both
seriously endanger our lives. Unfortunately, not eating them is much
easier said than done. Sugar is highly addictive and embedded in
most processed foods. Seed oils are not addictive but are embedded
in even more processed foods than sugar and can't be detected by
anything other than a chemical analysis.

This part of the book is a detailed guide to where to find sugar and the seed oils in most categories of food. It's tricky stuff if you want to keep eating processed foods, but it *is* possible. The simpler route to take, of course, is not to eat processed foods. If you restrict your shopping to the outer perimeter of the supermarket (i.e. if you 'shop the perimeter') you'll automatically avoid all added sugar and all seed oils. On the outer perimeter, you'll find fruit, vegetables, meat, milk, eggs and bread. The only place you need to exercise some caution is in the dairy cabinet, because most yoghurts contain added sugar, and of course that's where the seed-oil margarines live. But with those two 'gotchas' to observe, you can completely avoid the two primary causes of almost every chronic disease afflicting Australian society today.

That plan might be okay for some people – and I wish I were one of them – but the reality is that there are things in the inside aisles that I'd still like to eat. The good news is that with a bit of careful navigation, we can avoid both fructose and seed oils and still eat some processed foods. The bad news is that some categories of food are completely out – at least until the food manufacturers realise we're onto them and change their formulas, that is.

11. CUTTING OUT SUGAR – OR, MORE PRECISELY, FRUCTOSE

Sugar is highly addictive, a feature that's made it very popular with food processors, so before you can decide that it's no longer part of your life, you have to break your addiction. In *The Sweet Poison Quit Plan*, I mapped out (in excruciating detail) the steps needed to break a sugar addiction. If you're a fast learner, here's the potted summary (there, I'm just about to save you $30 – aren't I nice?).

Breaking your sugar addiction

There are five steps you have to take:

1. **Have the right attitude.** If you treat this as an exercise in deprivation, you'll never succeed. You're ridding yourself of a dangerous toxin and this step asks you to perform the attitude adjustment you'll need to get through the remaining steps.

2. **Eliminate habits associated with eating sugar.** Believe it or not, it is possible to enjoy a movie without a litre of soft drink for

company. This step asks you to document your sugar habits and create strategies for keeping the habit but getting rid of the sugar.

3. **Eliminate sugar from your food supply.** You'll never break an addiction if your kitchen is full of the addictive substance.

4. **Withdraw from sugar.** Intentionally and purposefully eat the last mouthful of sugar you'll ever touch in your life. Withdrawing from sugar is exactly the same as withdrawing from an opioid such as nicotine. You'll experience a withdrawal period, but when that ends you'll no longer be attracted to sugar in any form.

5. **Restock and get ready for the rest of your life.** Your home needs to be a sugar-free oasis for you and your family. You need to refill your cupboards with sugar-free food, so you're never tempted to become re-addicted. Once an addict, always an addict, and the smallest dose could take you back to that place.

In this book I'll focus on steps 3 and 5 (identifying the sugar and replacing it), but if you want more detail on the other steps, it might be worth picking up a copy of *The Sweet Poison Quit Plan* after all.

Avoiding fructose

The active ingredient in sugar, from an addiction point of view, is fructose. Thanks to the marvels of modern food production, fructose is now embedded in almost every single food item on the supermarket shelf. Quitting fructose is far harder than quitting nicotine – imagine how hard it would be stop smoking if everything you ate or drank contained the addictive ingredient.

You still have an addiction to fight, but before you even get that far you've got to pick your way through a minefield of fructose-filled foods. There are, however, some big food categories that anyone giving up fructose should absolutely avoid:

- Confectionery, ice-cream and bikkies (I know you knew that already, but just in case you forgot)
- Flavoured drinks – not just soft drinks; this includes juice and flavoured milk ('flavour' is usually just a euphemism for 'added sugar')
- Breakfast cereals
- Condiments (barbecue sauce, for example, has more sugar than chocolate sauce)
- Muesli bars
- Flavoured yoghurts
- And, of course, anything you add to food, such as table sugar, spreads and honey.

Avoid those foods and you'll have skipped 90 per cent of the fructose you're likely to encounter in a day. Obviously there are exceptions. For example, you can eat natural yoghurt (but you'd better get used to the sour taste) and you can eat porridge and most other unflavoured oat cereals. But the reality is that unless you restrict yourself to the exceptions I outline in the next section, the only way you'll eat many of the items above will be if you make them yourself.

The sugar exceptions – low-fructose processed foods

In each of the highly processed food categories outlined above, there are exceptions to a complete ban. Some foods are either very low in sugar altogether or are sweetened with dextrose rather than sugar (sucrose) or fructose. Dextrose is just another name for glucose, our natural fuel source. Our brain cannot run on anything other than pure glucose, and every carbohydrate and protein not used to build stuff is converted into glucose so we can use it for energy. We're perfectly adapted to control how much glucose we eat, and our appetite-control system will accurately monitor every calorie of glucose we ingest. For the recovering sugarholic, glucose is the perfect substitute for sugar. When your diet includes sugar, dextrose will taste a lot like flour, but once your palate adjusts after sugar withdrawal, it will taste like you remember sugar tasting.

Sweets

They're not easy to find, but some lines of confectionery are made from dextrose. They're usually sherbet-like lollies, often made into lollipops or little hard circles or rolled into a tube. Nestlé even makes Gobstoppers, which are sweetened only with dextrose. All of these sweets are traditionally on the sour or bland side, but to fructose-free kids and their parents they're a fantastic treat. Listed below are some of the fructose-free sweets I've found, but I keep finding more. Eagle-eyed shoppers can probably find something like these lollies in their local supermarket:

- Nestlé Wonka Gobstoppers – Chewy or Longlasting
- Mike & Jack Groovy Candy Rolls
- Mike & Jack Groovy Lollipops
- Glucodin tablets.

Of course, you can also make treats yourself. Most dessert, biscuit and cake recipes can be adjusted by taking out the sugar and putting in glucose (dextrose). It isn't always a one-for-one swap, but a few trial-and-error batches should allow you to sort out a recipe. If you'd rather not muck around, there's a bunch of recipes for such things in *The Sweet Poison Quit Plan*.

You won't be surprised to find that ice-cream is off the shopping list. Even a small bowl (200 grams) of the very best ice-cream still delivers two teaspoons of sugar, as well as several artificial sweeteners. And one of the sweeteners (sorbitol) is essentially metabolised as fructose anyway (for comprehensive information on artificial sweeteners, see my book *The Sweet Poison Quit Plan*). You'll be pleased to discover that ice-cream homemade using glucose is almost identical to ice-cream made from sugar.

Soft drinks

Drinking sugar is the single most efficient way to get it inside you. Truly vast quantities can be consumed without a second thought. Sweetened drinks are a fructose expressway to your bloodstream. The average child can down a small glass of apple juice (250 ml) in less time than it took you to read this sentence. By doing that, they're consuming the juice of three to four large apples. It would take my kids most of the morning to eat three large apples, but they can suck up the juice in an instant. You could drink a large apple juice and eat a full and hearty meal, but try eating the six large apples that produced the juice and see how far you get with the meal. A single 600 ml bottle of Coca-Cola (or just about any fizzy drink) will deliver about 66 grams of sugar (33 grams of fructose).

It's much easier to say which drinks are allowed than to specify the rest. The only drinks you should have in your cupboard or fridge are unflavoured water and unflavoured milk. It doesn't matter whether the milk is low-fat or regular, but research on low-fat products suggests you're much better off with the high-fat version (see Chapter 9). If you prefer your water with bubbles, then by all means have unflavoured mineral water or soda water.

If, after reading the section on artificial sweeteners in my book *The Sweet Poison Quit Plan*, you're still quite happy to drink diet soft drinks, then they can stay as well. When I was going through withdrawal, I desperately needed artificially sweetened drinks. I drank them when I went shopping, when I went to the movies, when I ate out and when I drank alcohol – and even when I was out but not drinking alcohol. I wouldn't have got through withdrawal without them, and if you're as big a user as I was, neither will you. The interesting thing is that after withdrawal, you won't hanker after artificially sweetened drinks. Once you've lost your desire for sweetness, these drinks will seem like strange-tasting substitutes for water. When fizzy drinks lose their addictive kick, there's not much to recommend them, especially if they also taste oddly metallic, which most artificially sweetened drinks do once your palate adjusts.

All other juices, soft drinks and flavoured milks are out of bounds. It doesn't matter whether the Dalai Lama hand-squeezed the juice next to a mountain spring or you buy it in a bottle, it's still just sugar and water, and it needs to go. Some people object to me describing juice as 'soft drink without the fizz'. They usually cite the nutrients in juices as a reason to keep drinking them, but the research doesn't back up their position. The primary nutrients in most juices are vitamins A and C, but there's no suggestion that supplementing with those vitamins is of any benefit to the average member of Western society (see Chapter 4). And, of course, there's nothing you'll get from a juice that you wouldn't also get from the fruit from whence it came. So, if you're utterly convinced that your life will be poorer without the nutrients likely to be found in a glass of orange juice, then eat the orange instead. This way, not only will you get the nutrients, you'll also get the fibre.

Sports drinks and their less sporty cousins 'vitamin waters' and 'energy drinks' are all sweetened with sugar and must be avoided. They generally contain slightly less sugar than soft drinks, but they still carry a significant sugary punch. One important exception may become very useful as you try to wean yourself off fructose – Lucozade Original (and only the original) is sweetened with pure glucose instead of sugar (but all the other Lucozade flavours are sweetened with sugar). If you're over 40, you'll probably remember your mother offering you Lucozade when you were sick. It tastes like a not-so-sweet lemonade and you can still buy it in the sports drink section of the supermarket. If you're attempting to take children on this sugar-free ride with you, it might be worth getting some Lucozade Original – when we took off on this path our kids enjoyed it as an occasional treat.

Soy milk and other milk substitutes

Soy milks are primarily created for lactose-intolerant people (lactose is the sugar in cow's milk). Most baby mammals, including humans, are adapted to survive on lactose when they're young, but about 70 per cent of the world's adult human population are lactose-intolerant and cannot digest lactose or use it for energy production. As they reach adulthood, these people lose the ability to manufacture the enzyme that chops lactose into its constituent galactose and glucose. People with ancestry in northern Europe, the Middle East and India (the places where people have the longest association with domesticated cattle) are more likely to continue to make the enzyme and to drink and eat milk products comfortably into adulthood. For everybody else, the products pass straight through the digestive system, which is why a primary symptom of lactose-intolerance is diarrhoea.

To make soy milk taste like milk, the manufacturers generally add sugar – cane sugar rather than lactose. This immediately removes soy milk from the list of acceptable drinks if you want to break your sugar addiction. And even if you weren't worried about the sugar content of soy milk, research shows that the unfermented soy it's made from materially harms our ability to use iodine (see Chapter 5).

How much sugar would you like in your milk?

Here's the sugar content of a small glass (250 ml) of some popular Australian soy milks (1 teaspoon of sugar is 4.2 grams):

Soy milk brand	Grams of sugar per 250 ml	Teaspoons of sugar per 250 ml
Vitasoy (original)	8.7	2.1
Bonsoy	5.5	1.3
Sanitarium So Good (regular)	5	1.2
Australia's Own Organic	5	1.2
So Natural (original)	4	0.95
Soya King	2.5	0.60

Eliminating soy milk doesn't mean that milk is completely off the menu if you're lactose-intolerant, however. Rice milk, which is usually made from brown rice, is normally sweet enough without added sugar. The sweetness in most rice milk varieties is generated by an enzymatic process that turns the long chains of glucose molecules (or starch, which is what rice largely is) into sugars, especially glucose. Some rice milk varieties may still be sweetened with sugar, so take a close look at the ingredients list to make sure none has been added. The label will say it's about 4 per cent sugar, but this is normally just glucose. The ingredients list should consist of water, rice, oil and salt, but no sugar.

Increasingly, enzyme-treated cow's milks, such as Paul's Zymil, are becoming available for the lactose-intolerant. The enzyme for chopping up lactose is introduced into these milks during the manufacturing process. This means the lactose comes pre-digested as galactose and glucose, and lactose-intolerant people can once again drink milk with the rest of us.

Powdered drinks

Powdered drinks are sold as food for toddlers, healthy afternoon snacks for teenagers and diet drinks for adults. All contain significant amounts of fructose and must be avoided.

By toddler food, I mean formulas for children older than 12 months. In Australia and New Zealand, formulas for children under 12 months are prohibited by law from containing sucrose (cane sugar). This is not the case in other countries, particularly the United States, so pay careful attention to the labels for all formulas if you're reading this anywhere other than Australia or New Zealand.

Many toddler formulas used to have cane sugar added to make it easier to convince young children to drink what would otherwise be pretty unpalatable stuff. If you have young children and want to avoid turning them into sugarholics, you need to check the labels on toddler formulas – almost half the powder used to be pure sugar in some cases. There's now a concerted move by manufacturers to replace sugar with glucose in most toddler formulas. At the time of writing, the only Australian manufacturer still using sugar in toddler formula was Bellamy's, in their Organic Toddler Milk. (They use organic sugar, of course, but that doesn't mean it's chemically any different from plain old garden-variety sugar!) That may have changed by the time you're reading this, so check the label. If you see 'organic sugar' (or just 'sugar') on the ingredients list, then avoid it.

No self-respecting four-year-old would drink toddler formula, so the food manufacturers produce 'fun' powdered drinks instead. None of the restraint now being shown in the toddler market is evident in the milk-flavouring market. Powdered milk flavours all contain significant quantities of cane sugar and should all end up in the pile you're taking out to the bin.

Adults like powdered drinks, too. Flavoured coffee powders (and syrups) and diet shakes have become very popular in the last few years. Neither has a place in a recovering sugarholic's pantry. Flavoured coffees such as Nestlé's Coffee-Mate range can be about one-third sugar. Diet shakes are even worse. Most powdered diet-shake drinks are sweetened with pure fructose. A serving of Coca-Cola the same size as one of these reconstituted shakes contains about the same amount of sugar, but because Coke uses table sugar (only half fructose) rather than pure fructose, it might find itself in the unusual position of being the healthier alternative. You'd need to drink almost twice as much Coke to get the same amount of fructose as is in the average weight-loss shake.

It will sound strange and boring before you give up sugar, but now when I want a drink, I drink water or sometimes milk. And tea or coffee with milk but no sugar are both fine. If those options don't appeal to me, then I'm not thirsty and I don't need a drink. But the same thing doesn't apply to alcoholic drinks, which we all know we rarely drink because we're thirsty.

Alcoholic drinks

The alcohol in wine is created by fermenting the sugars in grape juice (glucose, fructose and sucrose). The alcohol in beer is fermented maltose (maltose is two molecules of glucose joined together). Alcohol (or, more technically, ethanol) is fermented sugar. A dry wine contains barely any of the original sugar, but a sweet wine such as a botrytis or dessert wine still contains significant amounts of sugar – on average, they're about 5 per cent fructose. You can keep the dry wines, beers and spirits, but you need to toss out the dessert wines, ports, sweet sherries, liqueurs and mixers (unless they're diet mixers).

The other important thing to know about alcohol is that it, too, is metabolised very quickly to fat. Indeed, ethanol is almost as efficient as sugar at being converted to circulating fat. The chemical pathways are slightly different, but the creation of fat is still a direct outcome of alcohol consumption. When you're a sugarholic and a drinker, this can compound the problems relating to sugar consumption. You'll get fatter quicker and you'll accelerate towards all the diseases related to being overweight at a much greater rate. This is because you're layering occasional fat-creating alcohol consumption on top of minute-by-minute fat-creating fructose consumption.

Bear in mind, however, that although alcohol is not part of a sugar addiction, it is of course addictive in its own right. And one thing more recent studies have shown is that rats have a propensity to swap one addiction for another. You'll need to guard against the possibility of jumping out of the sugarholic frying pan and into the alcoholic fire.

Once you've eliminated fructose from your diet, the occasional alcoholic drink won't do any significant damage, and some research suggests it can actually assist arterial health. In this way, alcohol consumption is similar to eating whole fruit: the occasional piece won't hurt in an otherwise fructose-free diet and it will probably do some good. If, however, you were to consume alcohol at the rate you previously consumed fructose (up to 100 grams per day – which equates to approximately 20 standard drinks per day), then you won't have improved your lot at all. Even if there are slightly fewer ways to die from alcoholism than sugar, I don't regard this as a step forward. You should aim to have no more than one standard drink (5 grams of ethanol) per day once you've gone fructose-free.

Breakfast cereals

Before World War II, breakfast cereals were only eaten by people as a 'digestive aid'. If you were having a little trouble keeping things moving downstairs, then the doctor would suggest you consider cereal for breakfast rather than your usual lamb's fry or mutton chops. Needless to say, the breakfast-cereal market wasn't exactly going gangbusters. Competing with a cooked breakfast would always be a struggle for cereal makers if the only thing they had going for them was a swift passage.

The war changed many things but perhaps the biggest changes were those associated with the mass entry of women into the work-force. Traditional gender roles were thrown out and women were encouraged to take over the jobs previously dominated by men. When the men returned from the front, the women often stayed at work. With both adults in the house frequently working at least some of the time, the cooked breakfast quickly became a week-end luxury. You didn't have to hit a manufacturer over the head with a cereal box for them to recognise a real market opportunity. The range of cereals quickly blossomed and the ease of preparation became a major theme in breakfast-cereal advertising. But the real leap forward didn't happen until almost the end of the 1940s.

In 1949, a US cereal company called Post created the first cereal targeted at children. Sugar Crisp was sold as the delicious treat kids could have for breakfast or straight out of the box for a snack. Sugar was unabashedly the primary ingredient, and the sugar arms race began in earnest. Kellogg's jumped on the bandwagon in 1953 with Sugar Smacks (56 per cent sugar), quickly followed by Apple Jacks (48 per cent sugar) and Froot Loops (42 per cent sugar).

The kids raised on sugar cereals in the 1950s became the parents of the 1970s and 1980s. They'd been trained to look for cereals that tasted sweet, and the manufacturers of adult cereals were happy to oblige. Almost all cereals now sold in Australia contain significant amounts of sugar. The only cereals that contain even remotely acceptable levels of sugar are variations on unflavoured oats and wheat biscuits, provided, of course, you don't add sugar or honey yourself. One good alternative, especially in winter, is unflavoured porridge oats.

Sauces, chutneys and relishes

Condiments, by which I mean sauces and flavourings designed to be added to food after serving, are very dangerous territory for the recovering sugarholic. There's more sugar in barbecue sauce (55 per cent) than in chocolate topping (43 per cent). The reason barbecue sauce doesn't taste as sweet is that it's also loaded with salt to balance out the sweet taste.

Sauce	Sugar content
barbecue	48–55%
hoi sin	50%
steak	45%
sweet chilli	43–49%
brown (for example, HP)	26%
Ketchup	25%
Worcestershire	15–36%
tomato	21–36%
apple	15%
tartare	6–10%
fish	6%

laksa	5%
taco	1.5%
soy	1%
Tabasco	0
Chutney or relish	
fruit chutney	29–39%
gherkin relish	31%
barbecue relish	24%
tomato chutney or relish	18%
corn relish	17%
salsa	7–9%
pesto	2–5%

For some reason, this sort of condiment excites the creative bones in the food manufacturers, and the particular flavours and constitutions of each chutney or relish change quite frequently. So, if you're just ducking quickly into the condiments section for a pesto, check the label first. If you see more than 5 per cent sugar, put it back and move on.

The news on mustard, however, is all good. The average mustard has no sugar or just a teeny bit if it's a wholegrain variety (around 2 per cent from the grains).

Mayonnaise and salad dressing

Mayonnaise divides neatly into two camps: the stuff you've previously been told not to eat (whole-egg mayonnaise) because it contains the dreaded eggs, and the stuff I'm going to tell you not to eat now (the rest). Whole-egg mayonnaise is very low in sugar – most brands are less than 2 per cent sugar and quite a few are zero. The only one you need to watch out for is Praise's reduced-fat whole-egg mayo, which is 13 per cent sugar. Non-egg-based mayos marketed as 'traditional mayonnaise' have around 8.5 per cent sugar in the normal-fat versions and up to 21 per cent sugar in the reduced-fat versions, so avoid them at all costs. But if you're a mayo fan, you still need to tread carefully. Most of the big-brand mayos are made from sunflower oil, one of the nastiest seed oils. Olive-oil-based versions do exist, such as Pukara Estate brand, but are usually sold at a premium and you'll need to hunt carefully. Of course, you could just make your own – there are about a million recipes for olive oil mayo on the web – you'll need to use light olive oil, but be aware that this means light in flavour, not fat.

Unfortunately, traditional mayo is used as the basis for commercial coleslaw, so you can expect a big serve of sugar and seed oil if you buy pre-made coleslaw from the supermarket. Besides, making your own with the kids is good fun (seriously). Just chop up a cabbage of your choice, mix in some grated carrot, then stir in (this is where the kids come in – using their hands) a lump of whole-egg mayo, and Bob's your uncle. I defy you or your sugar-munching friends to detect the difference, but it's almost – except for the carrot and cabbage – fructose-free and, if you've made your own mayo or shopped in the premium aisle, it's also seed-oil-free.

Salad dressings don't exactly qualify for confectionery status, but some are alarmingly high in sugar and most should be avoided.

Salad dressing	Sugar content
thousand island fat-free	19%
thousand island	17%
balsamic vinegar	15%
French fat-free	9–17%

French	7–13%
Italian or Caesar fat-free	10%
Italian or Caesar	5%
ranch	6%
lemon juice	2.5%
vinegar	0
olive oil	0

You might be surprised to find that balsamic vinegar has so much sugar. The reason is that balsamic vinegar is not actually vinegar at all but a reduction of the syrup of sweet wine grapes. True vinegar is made by further fermenting wine (the word 'vinegar' derives from the Old French *vin aigre*, which means 'sour wine'). In balsamic, the grape sugar is still there, while in vinegar, it's all been fermented (initially to ethanol and ultimately to acetic acid).

The best thing to put on salad is air. If that's not to your taste, then try combining some or all of the last three things on the list above with some chopped herbs or wholegrain mustard – it should do the trick and will be virtually sugar-free.

Muesli and snack bars

There are no good options in the muesli-bar aisle – they're all full to the brim with sugar and most of them make the confectionery aisle look like the health-food section. Move along, there's nothing to see here.

Yoghurt

Yoghurt is a trap for new players. For the longest time, I purchased yoghurt on the understanding that when the label said 'no added sugar', that meant no added sugar. I eventually discovered that this is not exactly true. I was buying the Jalna range of fruit yoghurts because they were emblazoned with that phrase, but when the slogan suddenly changed to 'no added cane sugar', the red lights started flashing. Peering closely at the ingredients list, I found that there was indeed no cane sugar, but 'fruit juice extract' was pretty high on the list.

Fruit juice extract or concentrate is just another phrase that can be translated to 'sugar'. Sugar molecules are no less dangerous because they were once part of a piece of fruit rather than sugar cane. When I looked at an old yoghurt container, with the original 'no added sugar' terminology, I discovered, to my despair, that all the ingredients were the same. The only change was the (probably legally inspired) insertion of the word 'cane' into the proud boast on the front of the label. I was aghast. I'd been feeding my kids this stuff believing it to be sugar-free and it was nothing of the sort. No wonder they gobbled it up like it was ice-cream!

In its natural state, yoghurt is extremely tart. If what you're eating is anything other than sour-tasting, then it's been sweetened with something – either sugar, pure fructose (often described as 'concentrated fruit juice' on the label) or an artificial sweetener. Like milk, yoghurt contains lactose, so you need to deduct 4.7 grams per 100 grams to work out the fructose content. So, for example, you might notice that Jalna Biodynamic Fat Free is 4.7 per cent sugar (just like full-fat milk), but all of this would be lactose, so you can treat it as fructose-free and therefore safe to eat.

Spreads

Nestled near the bread in most supermarkets, you'll find things to spread on it (who says shopkeepers aren't smart?). There's almost nothing worth buying from this section, and the recovering sugarholic should avert their eyes as they pass through on their way to the perimeter. But just for fun, in the table below I've listed the average sugar content of the types of things you're likely to find in the spreads section.

Spread	Sugar content
honey	82%
fruit jams and conserves	65%
hazelnut spreads	55%
low-sugar jams and conserves	30–40%
peanut butter with honey	20%
peanut butter (salted)	9%
peanut butter without added salt	5.5%
Vegemite	2.2%

Vegemite is, thankfully, an acceptable spread – one 20 gram serve contains about 0.44 grams of sugar. If you're not a fan of Australia's national dish, then no-added-salt peanut butter might be worth considering were it not for the fat profile of peanut oil. But cream cheese spread is also an option – the 2.1 per cent sugar is all lactose, so it's effectively zero per cent fructose.

Everything else on the list should be a no-go zone for you. Honey is often sold as the 'natural alternative' (although it's not clear what it's an alternative to), but it doesn't matter if honey has been hand-farmed by your neighbour's grandad, it's still likely to be in the 80 per cent range for total sugars (and 40 per cent for fructose). Jams and conserves are also chock-full of sugar and must be avoided. And no matter how many ads you see testifying to the health benefits of chocolate hazelnut spreads, they're simply spreadable chocolate bars.

If Vegemite or cheese spread doesn't appeal, try one of my kids' favourites – avocado. Fresh avocado smeared on toast is a delicious spread, and you can liven it up with a little salt, pepper and maybe even a squeeze of lemon. Avocado is very high in fibre and has almost no fructose. As spreads go, it doesn't come any better.

12. CUTTING OUT POLYUNSATURATED FATS (SPECIFICALLY SEED OILS)

As strange as it might sound, avoiding seed oils is significantly more difficult than avoiding sugar. At least we can taste sugar. If a food tastes sweet it either contains sugar or an artificial sweetener, so even if we can't see a label (because we're in a restaurant, say), we've got a fair old clue that the food might be a problem. But to our tastebuds, a fat is a fat. We have no way of knowing by taste or consistency whether the fat is polyunsaturated or not.

We can only make two kinds of fat, saturated and monounsaturated. This is why 97 per cent of the fat in our body is one or other of those two types of fat. The other 3 per cent should be the polyunsaturated fats we get from our diet, the so-called essential fatty acids (essential because we need them and we can't make them). The two polyunsaturated fatty acids our bodies can't manufacture are linoleic acid (LA, an omega-6 fatty acid) and alpha-linolenic acid (ALA, an omega-3 fatty acid). They're both 18 carbons long. We need them to manufacture the hormone-like molecules we use to control many of our systems (mainly inflammation or immunity) and as messengers

221

in our central nervous system. But we only need a maximum of 3 per cent (and perhaps as little as 1 per cent) of the calories we consume to be made up of these essential fatty acids. And, as with most things in our body, we need the balance to be just right. If we have just the right amount of both, then things hum along. But if we push the balance between them out or have too many of them in total, we start to encounter the problems I set out in chapters 9 and 10.

Before the invention of agriculture and the introduction of seed-based foods into our diet, we probably consumed polyunsaturated fats in the ratio of one omega-6 to one omega-3. But for the 10 000 or so years between the invention of agriculture and the beginning of the industrial revolution (in the early 1800s), we appear to have done well on a ratio of about two omega-6 to one omega-3.

Omega-3 and omega-6 fatty acids

While most of us are getting just enough omega-3 ALA, we're now all getting vast amounts of omega-6 LA if we eat polyunsaturated seed oils or anything made with them – which is an awful lot of things.

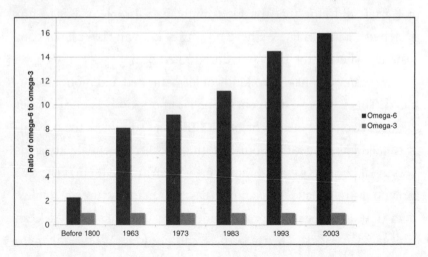

Ratio of omega-6 to omega-3 polyunsaturated fats over time for the UK population. We're a long way from the pre-seed-oil ratio of two to one.

Surveys into such things are pretty thin on the ground in Australia (or at least I didn't find any), but I've graphed some good recent data from the UK opposite. I don't think it's too big a stretch to suggest that in Australia we're probably tracking along a similar path to Britain. If that's the case, we're currently hovering around a ratio of 20 omega-6 to one omega-3 (in other words, 10 times the ratio of a mere 200 years ago).

Observations like this are the reason we're implored to take omega-3 supplements (fish oils and linseed/flaxseed oils). The thinking is that we can't reduce our polyunsaturated-fat intake because the alternative is animal fat and that's theoretically deadly, but most sources of polyunsaturated fats are very high in omega-6 and have virtually no omega-3. Therefore the obvious (they think) solution to the problem is to increase our consumption of omega-3. The theory is that then at least we might get our ratio of omega-6 to omega-3 back to what it should be.

It's a futile effort, because at current omega-6 consumption levels (about 10 per cent of calories) an adult male would need to consume about 14 grams of omega-3 oil a day. This is the amount in half a kilogram of north Atlantic salmon, three-quarters of a kilogram of herring, 6 kilograms of cod or 47 standard fish-oil or flaxseed-oil supplement pills. Even if we could successfully consume that much every day, we'd be significantly increasing our polyunsaturated-fat consumption. Yes, the ratio matters, but so does the amount. We don't need any more than 3 per cent of our diet to come from polyunsaturated fats (and of that, only a maximum of two-thirds should be omega-6). In Australia our polyunsaturated-fat intake is currently bobbing around above the 10 per cent level (largely omega-6 fats). If we actually tried to bring that back into balance by upping our consumption of omega-3 fatty acids, then 15–20 per cent of our calories would have to come from a source that science says is likely to be a major player not only in the in development of cancer (see Chapter 10), but also of heart disease (see Chapter 9).

The reason the amount of omega-6 we're consuming has got so large so quickly is pretty simple. As I illustrated in Chapter 8, the animal fats we eat are being progressively replaced with cheaper (and 'healthier', but most importantly cheaper) seed oils. It's now almost impossible to buy a deep-fried food in Australia cooked in anything other than a seed oil. The big-brand fast-food joints (such as McDonald's and KFC) use canola–sunflower blends, but even the corner fish and chipper is likely to be using 'vegetable oil'. This could be a blend of soy and sunflower oils (which are to be avoided) or it could be palm oil.

Palm oil

Although palm oil has a relatively low polyunsaturated-fat content (about 10 per cent), it's all omega-6, so I recommend you keep it to a minimum, to avoid spoiling your balance of omega-6 and omega-3 fats. But an even more important reason to avoid it has much more to do with the health of orangutans and natural rain-forest than humans.

Palm oil is obtained from the fruit of the African oil palm tree. These palm trees (which are more like bushes, really) are grown in massive plantations in equatorial regions (largely Indonesia and Malaysia). Demand for palm oil is accelerating enormously. Food manufacturers, particularly in India and China, want to use it because it can be labelled as a vegetable oil, but because it has high saturated-fat content, it behaves like lard in the fryer. Now that manufacturers are no longer able to hydrogenate seed oils (because that creates trans fats), palm oil is a great alternative. It allows them to say their product is made using vegetable oil, even though in real-ity it's very high in saturated fat.

From a biochemical perspective, I wouldn't mind that, but the problem is that in order to grow the palms, large tracts of native forest have to be destroyed. And in those forests live the last remaining members of several endangered species, including orangutans. If the market continues to grow at its current rate, it's likely that orangutans will be extinct within 20 years. And that's reason enough for me to avoid palm-oil-based products.

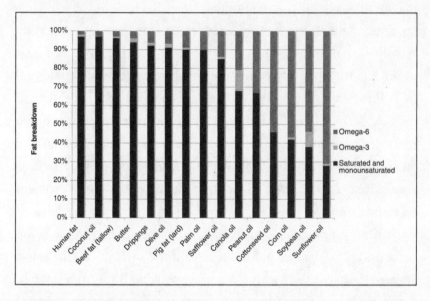

The fat profile of various fats and oils arranged from best (*left*) to worst (*right*). Anything to the right of (and including) palm oil contains too much omega-6 polyunsaturated oil. This is not a licence to eat humans!

Chips

The other bad news (and believe me, it was very bad news to me) is that unless you can locate someone who's prepared to fry your chippies in tallow or lard just like they used to, you need to give commercial fried foods a great big swerve.

The alternative, of course, is to make them yourself. And this is exactly what I've done. I acquired a deep-fryer (a large pot with a basket), 2 kilograms of dripping (much to the consternation of the folks at my local Woolies), a device that turns potatoes into chips (you know, the kind of thing you see demonstrated on very late-night tellie) and of course a bunch (or is it a herd?) of potatoes. Now when the kids and I want chips, I make 'em myself. That involves chippifying the potatoes, pre-frying them at a lower heat for five minutes, resting them for 10 minutes and then refrying them at maximum for another five minutes.

You could short-circuit the laborious chip-making process by buying frozen chips, which only need to be fried once at maximum. But the difficulty is that they're always pre-cooked in a seed oil before being snap-frozen. Not all are cooked in the same type of seed oil, so by carefully reading the labels you can narrow it down to the least harmful ones. Canola oil doesn't have enough saturated fat, but it's the only seed oil whose omega-6 to omega-3 ratio is about right (2:1) and you'll be correcting the saturated-fat problem to some extent by finishing the process in animal fat. So I'd seek out frozen chips cooked in canola oil rather than sunflower oil (as most are). If you've got the time and the inclination, the safest way to do it is to start with a whole potato and do it from scratch. I rather suspect that if you have anywhere near as many kids as me (six), then everybody might get much fewer chips than they're used to.

Reading the label

In Australia, a manufacturer need provide no more detail on a label about the oil used than the words 'vegetable oil' in the list of ingredients. What they really mean is 'seed oils', 'nut oils' or 'tropical fruit oils', but they're not required to spell that out. Vegetable oil on the label could be anything in the packet, but if it's canola oil (which is usually slightly more expensive and considered to be 'healthy'), they'll generally make a bit of a song and dance about it. If the product has a Heart Foundation Tick, and it says 'vegetable oil' on the label, then it's likely to be canola oil. If the product contains olive oil, the manufacturer will definitely say so. It's so (relatively) expensive they'll want you to know it's there. If the product contains soy oil, they'll usually say 'vegetable oil [contains anti-oxidants]' or something similar.

Margarine-makers feel the seed basis of their product is a selling feature, so they'll often say exactly which oil is being used (normally a blend of canola and sunflower). All are extremely bad choices, except for the rare few that only use olive oil.

If the label just says 'vegetable oil' assume the worst – that it's palm, soy or sunflower oil – and avoid it.

Crisps, biscuits and breads

Unfortunately, deep-fried foods are not the end of the story. Most crisps sold in Australia today are cooked in palm oil, although it will simply say 'vegetable oil' on the label. But some premium brands (such as Red Rock Deli) cook some varieties in olive oil. So if chippies are your thing, seek them out. They're not hard to find – they make a big deal of it – but they're usually significantly more expensive than garden-variety crisps.

And the horror doesn't end there. You won't be eating most biscuits because of the sugar content, but even cracker biscuits are full of 'vegetable oils'. Unless the label says exactly what the oil is (and most don't, probably because it's palm oil), I'd avoid them. Once again, some expensive brands are starting to do olive-oil-based versions, but these will be a bit exxy for the kids' lunchboxes. We've found we can do our own olive-oil equivalent of chips just by smearing oil over pita bread (one made without seed oils, such as Mountain brand), covering it with spices and popping it in the oven.

Most breads now include vegetable oil rather than the traditional lard, and it's usually, by the look of the anti-oxidant claims, soy oil or (sometimes) canola. It's there to make for a nice crispy crust. Look for breads with canola oil (such as Woolworths Home Brand) rather than breads that refuse to be specific about it. At least then you're getting a proper ratio of omega-6 to omega-3, even if there's too much polyunsaturated fat.

Baked and fried goods (this includes anything you're supposed to 'oven-fry' – which just means they've been pre-fried in seed oil and you're finishing them off in the oven) are the primary sources of seed oils in our diet, but they're creeping into other food categories as well, so you'll need to stay alert in the supermarket. Mixer sauces (you know, the sort of pre-made sauce that turns your chicken or mince into something flash) often include 'vegetable oils' and should be avoided, even if you weren't worried about their sugar content. And, of course, you'll also find vegetable oils in many breakfast cereals (for that crunch-in-the-mouth feel) except raw oats- and wheat-based products. Bizarrely, you'll also find vegetable oils in liquid versions of breakfast cereals, such as Sanitarium's Up & Go Range.

Beef and milk

Even if we stay away from commercial fried foods, crisps, crackers, cereals and simmer sauces, we'll still get more omega-6 than we should. Cattle are increasingly being fed on grains in preference to grass. A diet high in grains does to beef what it does to us: it increases both the amount and the proportion of omega-6 fatty acids. Grain-fed beef has an omega-6 to omega-3 ratio of 15:1 compared with the grass-fed ratio of about 2:1. We're not even completely safe with milk. Just as with humans, the fats a cow consumes are transferred into her milk. The milk of grain-fed cows has much higher polyunsaturated-fat levels and a much higher omega-6 to omega-3 ratio. If you get a choice about where your meat and milk (and of course cheese, butter, cream and yoghurt) come from, choose grass-fed over grain-fed every single time.

Seeds and nuts

Avoiding seed oils doesn't mean completely avoiding seeds and nuts. Oils are extracted from seeds and nuts using industrial processes under extreme pressure and heat. They're the edible-oil industry's version of juicing fruit (although it's a bit harder to get the 'juice' out) and they achieve exactly the same result. When we juice fruit we keep the bad bit (the fructose) and throw away the good bit (the fibre). When we extract seed and nut oils we keep the polyunsaturated fats and throw away the fibre. A cup of dried sunflower seeds will give you 10 grams of polyunsaturated oil (mostly omega-6) and an awful lot of fibre. A cup of sunflower oil would supply more than six times that much polyunsaturated fat (63 grams) and no fibre. Even so, you should choose seeds that are high in omega-3 (such as flaxseed) over seeds that are high in omega-6 (such as sunflower seeds), and eat nuts in preference to seeds because they have a significantly higher proportion of saturated and monounsaturated fat.

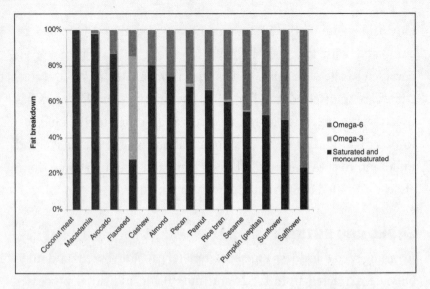

Fat breakdown of raw fruit, nuts and seeds arranged from best (*left*) to worst (*right*). Seeds in general (except flaxseed) should be avoided.

13. SO WHAT ARE WE ALLOWED TO EAT?

When you start listing things that aren't allowed (either because of their fructose or seed-oil content, or both), it's easy to start thinking you've just embarked on a diet of fresh air and not much else. Nothing could be further from the truth. Once you think about it, you'll realise that what you're left with is a diet very similar to what people ate before World War II.

A few things you can eat – I lack imagination so I'm sure you can come up with a lot more.

Breakfast	bacon (or sausages or steak) and eggs (if you leave the fat on you won't need cooking oil)	unflavoured porridge (oats)	wheat biscuits	toast (see spreads below)

Lunch	any burger you like (just hold the sauce)	sushi or sandwiches (without sugary spreads)	Asian, if you stay away from the high-sugar sauces	homemade meat pie (with homemade sauce)
Dinner	anything cooked in dripping, lard, tallow or olive oil	meat and three veg	homemade pizza (most commercial bases use seed oils)	Italian (if you make the sauce yourself)
Spreads	butter	Vegemite	cream cheese	avocado
Sandwich toppings	tomatoes and any other salad	meat	cheese	spreads (see above)
Snacks	olive-oil crisps or popcorn cooked in olive oil	nuts, cheese and (whole) fruit	homemade dextrose-based ice-cream, lollies, biscuits, cakes	unflavoured yoghurt with berries or pieces of fruit
Drinks	milk	water (with or without bubbles)	Lucozade Original	most alcohols (as long as the mixer is sugar-free)

We can eat any kind of meat, preferably grass-fed and preferably with the fat still attached. We can eat eggs and any dairy product. We can eat any fruit and vegetables as long as they're whole – in other words not juiced or dried. We can eat most kinds of bread. We can eat nuts and seeds, as long as they're whole and fresh. We can cook in animal fats, coconut oil or olive oil and we can spread butter on our bread. Is there actually any real food missing from that list?

232

Choose	Instead of
butter	margarine
whole milk and dairy	low-fat milk and dairy
grass-fed meat with fat attached	trimmed grain-fed meat
whole fruit and vegetables	dried, pureed or juiced fruit and vegetables
nuts	seeds
eggs	well, ah, not having eggs?

Don't worry about your fat intake

One of the things most people worry about when I suggest they eat full-fat anything is that just about everybody has told them to avoid fat. Once we stop eating sugar and our appetite-control system starts working properly again (see Chapter 6), the amount we can eat starts to fall fairly dramatically (and we lose weight). That, of course, means that we also end up eating less fat, but not because we're consciously counting calories or avoiding fat. Once you have a functioning appetite-control system, you simply can't eat that much fat and if you try (believe me, I've tried) you find yourself feeling physically ill well before you would have in your pre-sugar-free days. If we also ensure that the fat we eat closely matches our body's requirements (no more than 3 per cent polyunsaturated and of that preferably as little omega-6 and as much omega-3 as possible), then our body will function as intended and we'll avoid the damage that seed oils can inflict.

High-fat diets in history

I don't advocate people take up a very high-fat (90 per cent) diet (even if you could stand it). But those kinds of diets do exist, and even the people following them suffer no ill effects. The Ancient

Greeks knew that an effective treatment for epileptic fits was to starve the patient, and starvation remained an effective treatment option for much of human history after that. By the end of World War I, successful trials were being reported in mainstream medical publications. The problem with the theory was that it was only possible to starve someone for just so long (without the inconvenient side effect of death) and when they started eating again their seizures returned. This prompted research in the early 1920s looking for a way to get the benefits of starvation from a diet they could use for an extended period.

Researchers at the Mayo Clinic discovered that they could achieve the same effect just by ensuring the patient obtained their energy from ketones rather than glucose. Rollin Woodyatt had identified the presence of ketones as an alternative source of energy for the brain when patients were starved. Follow-up work discovered that ketones were only created when the body had exhausted all carbohydrates consumed and stored (in glycogen stores). The researchers found that if they completely restricted carbohydrate consumption, they could produce the same benefits for epileptics as starving them completely. The ketogenic diet was born. Patients were prescribed a diet with just enough protein to ensure that vital building and repair work continued (1 gram per kilogram of body weight) and almost no carbohydrates (10–15 grams per day – about a quarter of a slice of bread). The rest of the diet was fat.

With the seal of approval of the Mayo Clinic, the diet became very popular during the 1920s and 1930s and very successful at treating epilepsy. Then, in 1938, the first effective anticonvulsive drug was released and the ketogenic diet was consigned to the dustbin of history. It was much easier for neurologists to prescribe (and for patients to take) a drug than it was to ensure compliance with a difficult diet.

But that, thankfully, was not the end of the story. In 1994, the diet was featured on a US television show as a treatment used to control Charlie Abrahams' fits. Charlie was the two-year-old son of Jim Abrahams (a famous Hollywood writer, director and producer, responsible for such delights as *Airplane!*, *The Kentucky Fried Movie*, *Top Secret!*, *Ruthless People* and *Scary Movie 4*). Johns Hopkins Hospital had continued to offer the ketogenic diet to the few people who knew it existed, but by then it was generally regarded by the medical profession as a fringe therapy. Charlie's parents were desperate – his condition wasn't responding to the drugs. But using the diet, his epilepsy was controlled and his developmental progress resumed.

In 1997, Jim Abrahams made a hit movie about the experience, *First Do No Harm*, starring Meryl Streep, and the diet gradually clawed its way back into the mainstream of medical treatment for epilepsy, especially in childhood. Now a series of major trials of the diet has been published (two in 2009 alone) and the diet is being considered as a possible treatment for other neurological disorders, such as autism and brain tumours. It reduces seizure frequency by more than 50 per cent in half those who undertake treatment and by more than 90 per cent in a third of patients. About 20 per cent of children following the diet become completely free from seizures, and many are able to reduce their use of drugs or eliminate them altogether.

The treatment involves putting the patient on a diet very high in animal fats for years at a time. Naturally, researchers have been concerned about the potential for other adverse health outcomes in the children, and the question has been studied extensively. Some patients have increased blood-cholesterol levels, but these don't result in any health problems. The only known significant adverse effect is that around one in 20 develops kidney stones. This happens because the diet can occasionally create a condition called ketoacidosis, which results in abnormally high concentrations of calcium in the urine. The stones can be prevented by supplementing with potassium or increasing the amount of water the patient drinks (or both). But other than this, there have been no long-term health effects if appropriately treated. If left untreated, ketoacidosis can be fatal.

A typical ketogenic diet for a child

- **Breakfast** bacon and eggs (28 grams egg, 11 grams bacon, 37 grams of 36 per cent heavy whipping cream, 23 grams butter and 9 grams apple)
- **Snack** peanut butter ball (6 grams peanut paste and 9 grams butter)
- **Lunch** tuna salad (28 grams tuna, 30 grams mayonnaise, 10 grams celery, 36 grams of 36 per cent heavy whipping cream and 15 grams lettuce)
- **Snack** keto yoghurt (18 grams of 36 per cent heavy whipping cream, 17 grams sour cream, 4 grams strawberries and artificial sweetener)
- **Dinner** cheeseburger with no bun (22 grams minced beef, 10 grams cheese, 26 grams butter, 38 grams cream, 10 grams lettuce and 11 grams green beans)
- **Snack** keto custard (25 grams of 36 per cent heavy whipping cream, 9 grams egg and pure vanilla flavouring)

The ketogenic diet is well and truly at the extreme end of the fat-eating spectrum, and I don't suggest you try it unless it's been prescribed for the treatment of epilepsy. But it does provide a convenient emphasis of my point. High-animal-fat diets are not harmful. If a ketogenic diet is fine for a child for years at a time, why would anyone suggest that eating a diet consumed by our grand-parents (before we had a problem with diabetes, heart disease, cancer and weight gain) should cause any problems whatsoever?

Really, it's easy

The foods we can't eat are really just the foods invented in the last 100 years and peddled by the processed-food industry (and more lately endorsed by the health experts). They're the foods full of sugar and seed oils, most of which didn't exist at the start of last century. Avoiding them doesn't mean deprivation, but in some categories of foods (namely those entirely taken over by the processed-food industry) it does mean you might have to learn how to make it yourself.

What to avoid. Is it really that hard to give most of this stuff a swerve?

Breakfast	most packaged breakfast cereals (including mueslis)	flavoured oats	muesli bars	liquid breakfasts (such as Up & Go)
Lunch	anything fried at a national franchise	jam sandwiches	Asian with high-sugar sauces	anything else that can't be eaten without a slathering of high-sugar sauces

Dinner	anything fried in seed oil (including oven-bake frozen foods)	anything cooked in a simmer sauce	commercial pizza where the base is made with seed oil	Italian with commercial sauces
Spreads	margarine	jams	honey	Nutella
Snacks	dried fruit	most seeds (except flax)	commercial ice-cream, lollies, biscuits and cakes	flavoured yoghurt
Drinks	low-fat milk	soft drinks	fruit juices	dessert wines

You'll struggle to buy confectionery, cakes, lollies and ice-cream that aren't full of fructose or seed oils (or both). But CWA cookbooks were crammed with such stuff in days gone by. All we need to do is become a food-preparer rather than a food-assembler. The good news is that once we remove fructose from our diet, our desire for this category of food will wane significantly (all the more so if we have to learn to cook just to have a piece of cake). The bad news is that if you like fast food, you're going to discover it's quite a bit slower if you have to cut up a potato and wait for a deep-fryer to heat up.

If you can eat this way, your life will be immeasurably better. You'll lose weight, but you won't be on a diet (no willpower or exercise will be required). You'll materially reduce your risks of heart disease, stroke, type 2 diabetes, kidney disease and of course cancer, but you won't be taking drugs. And you'll experience a clarity of thought and consistency of mood you won't have imagined possible. Just break your addiction to sugar and keep it and seed oils out of your life. Easy. Good health!

Epilogue

Astute readers (and let's face it, if you've got this far, you're an astute reader) may have detected a theme or two to this book. Yes, there's the obvious theme that almost everything we're told to do about food is just plain wrong. Diets are a pointless band-aid that don't address the real reason we're fat (which is, of course, metabolic dysfunction brought on by sugar consumption). Exercise has its place, but that place is not in the bucket of weight-loss cures. Vitamins and minerals are important, but extracting them from food and taking just the extracts does nothing to help us at all. The only reason to avoid salt is if you've already stuffed up your kidneys with sugar. There's no reason to avoid dietary cholesterol and every reason to ensure you eat plenty of saturated and monounsaturated fat and virtually no polyunsaturated fat. And, of course, it's critically important to avoid fructose in your diet.

But the less obvious theme is that throughout the last 200 years, the health and food industries have been driven by just one thing – money. Their solution to every problem has been to add something to our diet (be it a drug or a vitamin) because then they have something to sell the afflicted punters. And there was even more to be made if governments could be convinced to add them to the food supply. Dosing us with supplements is always the preferred option for government.

The 'treat rather than prevent' habit runs into much deeper water than mere supplement-sellers. As soon as cholesterol was fingered as the 'cause' of heart disease (I'll give the drug companies the benefit of the doubt and assume they had nothing to do with Ancel Keys's anti-cholesterol campaign), the pharmaceutical giants were on the case with drugs – statins – that prevented us making cholesterol. Note that they didn't even attempt to look at our dietary levels, because they knew our cholesterol consumption had nothing to do with heart-disease outcomes. They've progressively convinced the health establishment to widen and further widen the definition of who should be taking statins until we're now almost certainly at the verge of having them added to our food supply. And make no mistake, very serious money is riding on our continued medication with statins – fully a quarter of legitimate drug money comes from them alone, and sales are growing very fast. There are billions of very good reasons to ensure we continue to believe that cholesterol is the problem, no matter what science now says or ever said.

Pharmaceutical and supplement companies are not the greatest beneficiaries of the misguided advice. The people making the most are the pushers of fructose and seed oils. Not the poor sugar, corn and canola farmers – they're just dispensable cogs in a brutal machine. In 2010, US farmers received just US$313 billion (19 per cent) of the US$1.6 trillion's worth of food sold in the US. The folks making the money are among the largest companies in the world today, and they barely existed a mere hundred years ago. Nestlé is the world's largest food company and the largest vendor of sugar-based products. PepsiCo is the largest food company in the United States. Unilever, created in 1930 by the amalgamation of British soap-maker Lever Brothers and Dutch margarine producer Margarine Unie, is the largest retailer of seed-oil-based products and ice-cream. And Kraft, now the proud owner of Cadbury chocolates, is slugging it out with Nestlé for world chocolate domination.

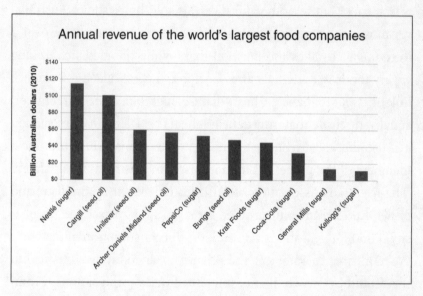

Behind the scenes the dollars are even bigger. Cargill, Archer Daniels Midland and Bunge jointly control the majority of the world's production of seed oils. Together they turn over more than US$200 billion a year (which makes Coke's lousy US$32 billion look like chicken feed). These very significant numbers provide very significant motivation to keep things just the way they are. For as long as these folks can keep our health authorities singing off their hymn sheets, there'll be no slow-down in the rivers of gold from seed oils and sugar.

The obvious question is why the status quo isn't being questioned by folks who should have our best interests at heart. None of the research I've mentioned in this book is secret. Most of it is recent and very little of it is controversial. So why isn't it causing consternation and soul-searching in the nutrition and heart-disease communities? The Australian Heart Foundation's Tick certification program completely ignores the sugar content of any food it endorses. It certifies Nestlé's Fruit Fix snack bar for children, which is 72 per cent sugar, on the basis that it's low in saturated fat. It gives a Tick to 44 of the 46 breakfast cereals sold by Nestlé in Australia, yet most of them are at least a quarter sugar and some are over a third sugar. It takes the position that 'While the evidence linking sugary foods with dental caries is strong, there is a lack of evidence linking sugar to diabetes, heart disease, high blood pressure, hyperactivity or inadequate nutrient intake'. The Dietitians Association of Australia, meanwhile, accepts corporate sponsorship from most members of the processed-food industry in Australia. It has stated: 'The Dietitians Association of Australia believes it is simplistic and unhelpful to blame sugar alone for such a complex issue [as obesity].' Both organisations also endorse the consumption of seed oils. We're all free to interpret the science in any way we see fit, but there's an obvious conflict of interest in these organisations recommending foods produced by the companies from which they accept money.

That kind of thing would be merely intriguing if most of what we're told we should and shouldn't eat didn't ultimately emanate from either or both of these entities. Nutrition advice untainted by the smell of food-industry money is almost impossible to obtain in Australia today. Even when you pay for a commercial diet, there's a good chance you're actually buying it from a card-carrying member of the food-processing industry. Sadly, it appears the barbarians are at the gate and our gatekeepers have been taken out to lunch.

I don't expect you to accept everything I say uncritically, either. For all you know, I'm sponsored by the butter industry or such like (I'm not). But if you read the 'Notes' section of this book carefully, you should at least be able to see where the information I've presented comes from and, if you wish, cross-check everything I say – isn't the interweb a wonderful thing?

There are no good reasons to consume fructose or seed oils. Both substances significantly degrade our ability to function as we are meant to and both substances materially increase our chances of an early and unpleasant death. But the good news is that both are easy to avoid. If you're happy to ignore any food introduced into our food supply since 1800, the job is done. If you'd still really prefer to eat from the centre aisles of the supermarket, you'll need to get your fructose- and seed-oil-spotting eye in. With a little knowledge, which I hope this book has passed on, and a little practice, there's no reason you can't skip past the health landmines laid for you by the processed-food industry.

Notes

Introduction The numbers on the reading habits of the medical profession come from 'Proliferations of Scientific Medical Journals: A Burden or A Blessing', *Oman Medical Journal* 25 (4), 311–14, October 2010, DOI: 10.5001/omj.2010.89.

PART 1: THE THINGS WE DO THAT MAKE NO DIFFERENCE TO OUR HEALTH

1. Why diets don't work

Counting calories Obviously the 25 calorie number is an arbitrary example based on the assumptions I state about how fast we gain weight. That being said, most of us tend to put on weight at a fairly steady rate after our teenage years and for most of us, the 25 calorie a day number will not be too far from the mark. I owe much of my thinking on calories to Gary Taubes (author of *Good Calories, Bad Calories*). We met in late 2010 and he told me his micro-calorie-counting analogy, my version of which is largely as set out in this section. I see that since then (in his latest book, *Why We Get Fat*) he's written it down. If you want a much more detailed explanation of how this all hangs together, then I can't recommend his books too highly.

How our bodies react to calorie restriction Keys's starvation study can be found at: Keys, A., Brozek, J., Henschel, A., Mickelsen, O. & Taylor, H. L. (1950) *The Biology of Human Starvation I–II*, University of Minnesota Press, Minneapolis, MN. Unfortunately, it's not available online. The abstract on the *Biggest Loser* was presented at the 71st Scientific Sessions of the American Diabetes Association and was entitled 'Greater Metabolic Adaptation Despite Fat-free Mass Preservation Following Dramatic Weight Loss Via Intensive Lifestyle Intervention Versus Bariatric Surgery'.

Do calorie labels work? The New York Study on calorie labelling is 'Calorie Labeling and Food Choices: A First Look at the Effects on Low-income People in New York City', *Health Affairs* 28(6): 1110–21, November/December 2009, DOI: 10.1377/hlthaff.28.6.w1110.

2. The weight-loss methods we try

The stats on how many of us are tubby come from the Australian Parliamentary briefing notes on obesity. Figures on how many folks are on a diet come from 'Prevalence of Attempting Weight Loss and Strategies for Controlling Weight', *JAMA* 282(14): 1393–94, 1999, DOI: 10.1001/jama.282.14.1393. And the amount we spend on weight loss comes from IBISWorld's report *Weight Loss Services in Australia: Market Research Report*.

Low-fat/low-calorie diets You can read the patents on the Weight Watchers formula for yourself. The 'old' one is US patent 6 040 531 and the new one is International Patent application WO 2010025422.

Do low-fat diets actually work? The Weight Watchers study is 'Weight Loss With Self-help Compared With a Structured Commercial Program', *JAMA* 289(14): 1792–98, 2003, DOI: 10.1001/jama.289.14.1792 and the Jenny Craig Study is 'Effect of a Free Prepared Meal and Incentivized Weight Loss Program on Weight Loss and Weight Loss Maintenance in Obese and Overweight Women', *JAMA* 304(16): 1803–10, 2010, DOI: 10.1001/jama.2010.1503. The research on what we can assume about people who drop out of studies like this is 'Evaluation of an Intensive Weight Control Program Using a Priori Criteria to Determine Outcome', *International Journal of Obesity and Related Metabolic Disorders* 16: 505–17, 1992, PMID: 1323547.

Does meal replacement actually work? The 2005 University of Pennsylvania Study is 'Systematic Review: An Evaluation of Major Commercial Weight Loss Programs in the United States', *Annals of Internal Medicine* 142: 56–66, 2005, PMID: 15630109.

Do low-carb diets actually work? The reason low-fat diets make us hungry is that they're generally high-carbohydrate diets. When we eat large amounts of carbohydrates, we stimulate insulin production and then (when the glucose is removed by the influx of insulin) stimulate glucagon, which makes us feel hungry. There's no equivalent of glucagon in our protein and fat appetite-control systems, so on high-fat or high-protein diets we tend to feel full or not-full, but we don't get hungry.

Studies on low-carb versus low-fat diets The 2003 study that compared low-carb with low-fat was 'A Randomized Trial of a Low-carbohydrate Diet for Obesity', *New England Journal of Medicine* 348: 2082–90, 2003.

What is the GI? The study that compared a low-GI diet to a low calorie diet is 'Effects of a Reduced-glycemic-load Diet on Body Weight, Body Composition, and Cardiovascular Disease Risk Markers in Overweight and Obese Adults', *American Journal of Clinical Nutrition*, 85(3): 724–34, March 2007.

Calorie-restriction diets really don't work Traci Mann's study is 'Medicare's Search for Effective Obesity Treatments: Diets Are Not the Answer', *American Psychologist*, 62(3): 220–33, Apr 2007, DOI: 10.1037/0003-066X.62.3.220.

Is weight-loss surgery an option? The study on the effectiveness of lap-band surgery is 'Cost-effectiveness of Surgically Induced Weight Loss for the Management of Type 2 Diabetes: Modeled Lifetime Analysis', *Diabetes Care* 32(4): 567–74, April 2009, DOI: 10.2337/dc08-1749.

3. Exercise won't help you lose weight, either

You can get your own personal copy of the Australian Sports Commission's annual report from their website. The 2009 version (the latest version at the time of writing) is available at ausport.gov.au/__data/assets/pdf_file/0005/377069/ERASS_Report_2009.pdf. The data on how much Americans spend on sports equipment comes from the Sporting Goods Manufacturers Association, 'the trade association of leading industry sports and fitness brands'.

How exercise got tied up with weight loss Jean Mayer died of a heart attack, aged 72, in 1993. Read his obituary at nytimes.com/1993/01/02/us/jean-mayer-72-nutritionist-who-led-tufts-dies.html?pagewanted=all&src=pm. His Indian study is 'Relation between Caloric Intake, Body Weight, and Physical Work: Studies in an Industrial Male Population in West Bengal', *American Journal of Clinical Nutrition* 4(2): 169–75, March 1956.

The truth about exercise The 2010 study is 'Fatness Leads to Inactivity, but Inactivity Does Not Lead to Fatness: A Longitudinal Study in

Children (EarlyBird 45)', *Archives of Disease in Childhood*, DOI: 10.1136/adc.2009.175927. And this is the American Heart Association review that found no compelling evidence for a link between obesity and exercise: acsm.org/AM/Template.cfm?Section=Home_Page&TEMPLATE=CM/HTMLDisplay.cfm&CONTENTID=7764. Lewis Newburgh's 1942 paper is simply called 'Obesity' and can be found at *Archives of Internal Medicine* 70(6): 1033–96, 1942.

Does regular exercise cause weight loss? The 2011 study is 'The Effect of Physical Activity on 18-month Weight Change in Overweight Adults', *Obesity* 19(1): 100–109, 2011, DOI: 10.1038/oby.2010.122.

4. Vitamins – don't waste your money

The information on what vitamins Americans are consuming comes from 'Dietary Supplement Use by US Adults: Data from the National Health and Nutrition Examination Survey 1999–2000', *American Journal of Epidemiology* 160 (4): 339–49, 2004. The Australian numbers come from 'Predictors of Dietary and Health Supplement Use in Older Australians', *Australian Journal of Advanced Nursing* 23(3): 26–32, 2006, and 'The Escalating Cost and Prevalence of Alternative Medicine', *Preventative Medicine* 35(2): 166–73, 2002. The data on dietary sources for each of the vitamins come from the exceedingly detailed databases maintained by the United States Department of Agriculture at ars.usda.gov/Services/docs.htm?docid=9673.

The discovery of vitamins: vitamin B1 You can read all about Christiaan Eijkman and Sir Frederick Hopkins on the Nobel Prize website at: http://nobelprize.org/nobel_prizes/medicine/laureates/1929/eijkman-bio.html and http://nobelprize.org/nobel_prizes/medicine/laureates/1929/hopkins.html

The discovery of vitamin C The British vitamin C experiments were republished in 'Medical Experiments Carried out in Sheffield on Conscientious Objectors to Military Service During the 1939–45 War', *International Journal of Epidemiology* 35(3): 556–58, 2006, DOI: 10.1093/ije/dyl020. And a great summary of the studies done after that is found in 'Human Requirements for Vitamin C and its Use in Clinical Medicine', *Annals of the New York Academy of Sciences* 92(1): 230–45, 1961, DOI: 10.1111/j.1749-6632.1961.tb46123.x. If you'd like to indulge in a little speculation about why humans no longer have the ability to make vitamin C, then 'Similar Functions of Uric Acid and Ascorbate in Man?', *Nature* 228: 868, 1970, DOI: 10.1038/228868a0 is definitely worth a glance.

Why we need sun If you'd like to know exactly how much sun you should get based on where you live, then 'Vitamin D Deficiency in Adults', *Australian Prescriber* 33: 103–106, 2010 (see australianprescriber.com/magazine/33/4/103/6), gives a city-by-city breakdown. The trials detecting an inverse association between sun exposure and heart disease and cancer are summarised in 'Prevalence of Cardiovascular Risk Factors and the Serum Levels of 25-hydroxyvitamin D in the United States', *Archives of Internal Medicine* 167(11): 1159–65, 2007, and 'Vitamin D Deficiency', *New England Journal of Medicine* 357: 266–81, 2007.

Do vitamins cure cancer? The 1981 review of animal studies that suggested vitamin A might be a cure for cancer is 'Can Dietary Beta-carotene Materially Reduce Human Cancer Rates?', *Nature* 290: 201–208, 1981, DOI: 10.1038/290201a0. The Finnish smokers trial is written up in 'Alpha-tocopherol and Beta-carotene Supplements and Lung Cancer Incidence in the Alpha-tocopherol, Beta-carotene Cancer Prevention Study: Effects of Base-line Characteristics and Study Compliance', *Journal of the National Cancer Institute* 88(21): 1560–70, 1996. And the US smokers trial is written up in 'Effects of a Combination of Beta-carotene and Vitamin A on Lung Cancer and Cardiovascular Disease', *New England Journal of Medicine* 334(18): 1150–55, 1996. The 1985 Chinese trial is reported in 'Nutrition Intervention Trials in Linxian, China: Supplementation with Specific Vitamin/Mineral Combinations, Cancer Incidence, and Disease-specific Mortality in the General Population', *Journal of the National Cancer Institute* 85(18): 1483–92, 1993. The 1994 folic acid trial is written up in 'Folic Acid for the Prevention of Colorectal Adenomas: A Randomized Clinical Trial', *JAMA* 297(21): 2351–59, 2007.

Is vitamin C a miracle cure? The 2007 Cochrane review can be found in 'Vitamin C for Preventing and Treating the Common Cold', *Cochrane Database of Systematic Reviews*, issue 3, article number CD000980, DOI: 10.1002/14651858.

The B-group vitamins and heart disease The results of the VITATOPS trial are available in 'B Vitamins in Patients with Recent Transient Ischaemic Attack or Stroke in the VITAmins TO Prevent Stroke (VITATOPS) Trial: A Randomised, Double-blind, Parallel, Placebo-controlled Trial', *Lancet Neurology* 9(9): 855–65, 2010.

Vitamins C and E and heart disease The study that shows vitamin C doesn't affect heart disease outcomes is 'Effect of Vitamin C Supplementation on Lipoprotein Cholesterol, Apolipoprotein, and Triglyceride Concentrations', *Annals* *of Epidemiology* 5(1): 52–59, 1995, and the one that shows it has no effect on death rates is 'Mortality in Randomized Trials of Antioxidant Supplements for Primary and Secondary Prevention: Systematic Review and Meta-analysis', *JAMA* 297(8): 842–57, 2007. The Physicians Health Trial is reported in 'Vitamins E and C in the Prevention of Cardiovascular Disease in Men: The Physicians' Health Study II Randomized Controlled Trial', *JAMA* 300(18): 2123–33, 2008.

Other vitamin 'cures' The vitamin K trial can be found at 'Vitamin K Supplementation in Postmenopausal Women with Osteopenia (ECKO Trial): A Randomized Controlled Trial', *PLoS Medicine* 5(10): 1–12, 2008, and the multivitamin study is 'Multivitamin Use and the Risk of Mortality and Cancer Incidence: The Multiethnic Cohort Study', *American Journal of Epidemiology*, 2011, DOI: 10.1093/aje/kwq447.

Folate and spina bifida The study that sets out the link between maternal folate consumption and neural tube defects is 'Prevention of Neural Tube Defects: Results of the Medical Research Council Vitamin Study', *Lancet* 338(8760): 131–37, 1991, and the paper that examined the changes wrought by mandatory supplementation is 'Spina Bifida and Anencephaly before and after Folic Acid Mandate – United States, 1995–1996 and 1999–2000', *Morbidity and Mortality Weekly Report* 53(17): 362–65, 2004.

Is folate good for the rest of us? The paper examining the trends in blood-folate concentration in the population as a whole since food supplementation in the US is 'Trends in Blood Folate and Vitamin B12 Concentrations in the United States, 1988–2004', *American Journal of Clinical Nutrition* 86(3): 718–27, 2007. The 2007 study of Americans older than 70 is 'Folate and Vitamin B12 Status in Relation to Anemia, Macrocytosis, and Cognitive Impairment in Older Americans in the Age of Folic Acid Fortification', *American Journal of Clinical Nutrition* 85(1): 193–200, 2007, and the 2006 study of postmenopausal women is 'Unmetabolized Folic Acid in Plasma Is Associated with Reduced Natural Killer Cell Cytotoxicity among Postmenopausal Women', *Journal of Nutrition* 136(1): 189–94, 2006. The 10-year study of 25 000 postmenopausal women is 'Folate Intake, Alcohol Use, and Postmenopausal Breast Cancer Risk in the Prostate, Lung, Colorectal, and Ovarian Cancer Screening Trial', *American Journal of Clinical Nutrition* 83(4): 895–904, 2006, and the 2007 study on the effects of folate on colorectal cancer risk is 'Folic Acid for the Prevention of Colorectal Adenomas', *JAMA* 297(21): 2351–59, 2007, DOI: 10.1001/jama.297.21.2351

How harmful is vitamin A? The large study linking vitamin A with birth defects is 'Teratogenicity of High Vitamin A Intake', *New England Journal of Medicine* 333: 1369–73, 1995, and the study showing the link with bone-density problems is 'Excessive Dietary Intake of Vitamin A Is Associated with Reduced Bone Mineral Density and Increased Risk for Hip Fracture', *Annals of Internal Medicine* 129(10): 770–78, 1998. The trial showing an increased risk of lung cancer in smokers who took vitamin A supplements is 'Effects of a Combination of Beta-carotene and Vitamin A on Lung Cancer and Cardio-vascular Disease', *New England Journal of Medicine* 334(18): 1150–55, 1996.

Why don't vitamin supplements work? The analysis of the studies that show lowered heart-disease risk for folks who eat their vegies is 'Fruit and Vegetable Consumption and Risk of Coronary Heart Disease: A Meta-analysis of Cohort Studies', *Journal of Nutrition* 136(10): 2588–93, 2006, and the one for cancer outcomes is 'Association between Fruit and Vegetable Consumption and Oral Cancer: A Meta-analysis of Observational Studies', *American Journal of Clinical Nutrition* 83(5): 1126–34, 2006.

Should vitamins be added to food? The PricewaterhouseCoopers report that lists the functional food players is 'Leveraging Growth in the Emerging Functional Foods Industry: Trends and Market Opportunities – 2009', pwc.com/us/en/transaction-services/publications/functional-foods.jhtml.

5. Salt and other minerals

Calcium and vitamin D The UK trial was reported in 'Oral Vitamin D3 and Calcium for Secondary Prevention of Low-trauma Fractures in Elderly People (Randomised Evaluation of Calcium Or vitamin D, RECORD): A Randomised Placebo-controlled Trial', *Lancet* 365(9471): 1621–28, 2005, and the 2004 systematic review appears in 'Calcium Supplementation on Bone Loss in Post-menopausal Women', *Cochrane Database of Systematic Reviews*, issue 1, article number CD004526, 2004, DOI: 10.1002/14651858.

Is salt bad for us? The 2008 study showing that low salt levels increase our risk of death is 'Sodium Intake and Mortality Follow-up in the Third National Health and Nutrition Examination Survey (NHANES III)', *Journal of General Internal Medicine* 23(9): 1297–302, 2008.

Chromium deficiency and sugar When we're deficient in a mineral, it's usually because we don't eat the foods containing it in sufficient quantities, but chromium deficiency is generally caused by us getting rid of more of it than we should. It's not that we're short of chromium in our diet, just that we get rid of way too much of it if we eat sugar. Three excellent papers on chromium and its relationship to sugar and insulin sensitivity are: 'Effects of Diets High in Simple Sugars on Urinary Chromium Losses', *Metabolism* 35(6): 515–18; 'Nutritional Factors Influencing the Glucose/Insulin System: Chromium', *Journal of the American College of Nutrition* 16(5): 404–10; and 'Elevated Intakes of Supplemental Chromium Improve Glucose and Insulin Variables in Individuals with Type 2 Diabetes', *Diabetes* 46(11): 1786–91, 1997.

Iodine deficiency and fructose The studies on the effect of iodine deficiency on the IQ of a newborn child are summarised nicely by UNICEF at ceecis.org/iodine.html. The USDA study on copper deficiency and fructose is 'Effect of Fructose or Starch on Copper-67 Absorption and Excretion by the Rat', *Journal of Nutrition* 116: 625–32, 1986, and the Russian research on the effect of copper on iodine status appears in 'The Effect of Copper on the Metabolism of Iodine, Carbohydrates and Proteins in Rats', *Fiziologicheskii Zhurnal* 36(2): 35–43, 1990. The article that discusses the current iodine-deficiency problems among Australian mothers is 'Iodine Deficiency in Australia: Is Iodine Supplementation for Pregnant and Lactating Women Warranted?', *Medical Journal of Australia* 192(8): 461–63, 2010.

PART 2: THE REAL CULPRITS: SUGAR AND POLYUNSATURATED FAT

6. Why we really gain weight – sugar

The notes for this chapter are intentionally thin on the ground because the chapter itself is really just a summary of what I've written in *Sweet Poison* and *The Sweet Poison Quit Plan*. If you really want to get among the detail, I suggest you start with *Sweet Poison* and follow the studies through from the 'Notes' section of that book. That being said, the few extra studies I've referred in this chapter are listed below.

Type 2 diabetes The University of California trial involving 32 people is reported in 'Consuming Fructose-sweetened, not Glucose-sweetened, Beverages Increases Visceral Adiposity and Lipids and Decreases Insulin Sensitivity in Overweight/Obese Humans', *Journal of Clinical Investigation* 119(5): 1322–34, 2009, DOI: 10.1172/JCI37385.

Kidney disease In an interview with Joel Gibson of *The Age*, printed on 18 September 2007, the Australian bottlers of Coca-Cola said they didn't know the source of a claim on their parent company's website that 'the Northern Territory has the highest per capita consumption rate of Coca-Cola in the world'. But a spokesperson for the local bottlers was paraphrased as saying, 'the soaring rates of diabetes and heart disease among the Northern Territory's Indigenous communities were made worse by products such as Coke and Fanta and the company had embarked on a campaign to wean Aboriginal people off sugary soft drinks.' The studies linking uric acid, kidney disease and hypertension are summarised succinctly in 'Is There a Pathogenetic Role for Uric Acid in Hypertension and Cardiovascular and Renal Disease?', *Hypertension* 41: 1183–90, 2003, DOI: 10.1161/01.HYP.0000069700.62727.C5. The 2008 Vienna University study is 'Elevated Uric Acid Increases the Risk for Kidney Disease', *Journal of the American Society of Nephrology* 19: 2407–13, 2008, DOI: 10.1681/ASN.2008010080. The 1989 USDA work on uric acid spikes caused by fructose is reported in 'Blood Lipids, Lipoproteins, Apoproteins, and Uric Acid in Men Fed Diets Containing Fructose or High-amylose Cornstarch', *American Journal of Clinical Nutrition* 49(5): 832–39, 1989. The schoolchildren study is 'Sugar-sweetened Beverages, Serum Uric Acid, and Blood Pressure in Adolescents', *Journal of Pediatrics* 154(6): 807–13, 2009, DOI: 10.1016/j.jpeds.2009.01.015, and the study on adults published in the same year is 'Sugary Soda Consumption and Albuminuria: Results from the National Health and Nutrition Examination Survey, 1999–2004', *PLoS One* 3(10): e3431, 2008.

Gout The large 2007 study is 'Soft Drinks, Fructose Consumption, and the Risk of Gout in Men: Prospective Cohort Study', *British Medical Journal* 336: 309, 2008, DOI: 10.1136/bmj.39449.819271.BE.

High blood pressure The recent human trial on reversing fructose-induced high blood pressure is reported in 'Combination of Captopril and Allopurinol Retards Fructose-induced Metabolic Syndrome', *American Journal of Nephrology* 30: 399–404, 2009, DOI: 10.1159/000235731.

Fructose and cancer The three large studies linking pancreatic cancer and sugar consumption are: 'Dietary Sugar, Glycemic Load, and Pancreatic Cancer Risk in a Prospective Study', *Journal of the National Cancer Institute* 94(17): 1293–1300, 2002; 'Consumption of Sugar and Sugar-sweetened Foods and the Risk of Pancreatic Cancer in a Prospective Study', *American Journal of Clinical Nutrition* 84(5): 1171–76, 2006; and 'Soft Drink and Juice Consumption and Risk of Pancreatic Cancer: The Singapore Chinese Health Study', *Cancer Epidemiology, Biomarkers & Prevention* 19: 447, 2010. The 2010 study that goes a long way to explaining the potential mechanism is 'Fructose Induces Transketolase Flux to Promote Pancreatic Cancer Growth', *Cancer Research* 70: 6368, 2010.

7. All about fats

I had to read a lot of textbooks about the biochemistry of fat to put this chapter together, but I won't bore you by listing them all. If, however, you're obsessed with the detail, then the best possible place to start is Mary G. Enig's magnificent book *Know Your Fats: The Complete Primer for Understanding the Nutrition of Fats, Oils and Cholesterol*, Bethesda Press, Silver Spring, Maryland, 2000. It might seem counterintuitive that a double bond is less stable than a single bond, and it certainly looks stronger the way it's drawn, but in chemistry bond strength and stability (or chemical reactivity) are not the same thing. The C-to-C double bond is stronger than the C-to-C single bond, but the electrons binding multiply bonded atoms are more vulnerable to attack by electron-seeking species (such as oxygen). Attack by an electron-seeker is a very different process from that of simply pulling the atoms apart.

8. Good fat, (very) bad fat

Cholesterol and atherosclerosis A great summary of Anitschkow's work has been published in 'Nikolai N. Anichkov and His Theory of Atherosclerosis', *Texas Heart Institute Journal* 33(4): 417–23, 2006, and if you're really keen (and can read German) his original publication is Anitschkow N. N. & Chatalov S. 'Über experimentelle Cholesterinsteatose und ihre Bedeutung für die Entstehung einiger pathologischer Prozesse', *Zentralblatt für Allgemeine Pathologie und pathologische Anatomie* 24: 1–9, 1913. The 1946 medical textbook is J. P. Peters and D. D. Van Slyke's *Quantitative Clinical Chemistry, Vol. 1: Interpretations*, Williams and Wilkins, Baltimore, 1931 (revised 1946). The 1950 human study that showed dietary cholesterol had nothing to do with heart disease is 'Diet, Serum Cholesterol and Coronary Artery Disease', *Circulation* 2: 696–704, 1950, DOI: 10.1161/01.CIR.2.5.696.

Keys's research into heart disease Keys's 1953 paper is 'Atherosclerosis: A Problem in Newer Public Health', *Journal of the Mount Sinai Hospital, New York* 20(2): 118–39, 1953. The problems with Keys's selective approach to the data were first pointed out in 'Fat in the Diet and Mortality from Heart Disease: A Methodologic Note', *New York State Journal of Medicine* 57(14): 2343–54, 1957. Keys's Seven Countries Study was published as a book entitled *Seven Countries: A Multivariate Analysis of Death and Coronary Heart Disease*, Harvard University Press, Cambridge, Massachusetts, 1980.

The role of drug companies The Lipid Research Clinics Coronary Primary Prevention Trial was published as 'The Lipid Research Clinics Coronary

Primary Prevention Trial Results: I. Reduction in Incidence of Coronary Heart Disease', *JAMA* 251(3): 351–64, 1984.

The truth about saturated fat The Framingham Heart Study has its own website – framinghamheartstudy.org – with a full list of all the results they've ever published. Dr William Castelli's quote appears in 'Concerning the Possibility of a Nut . . .', *Archives of Internal Medicine* 152(7): 1371–72, 1992. The Western Electric study was published as 'Diet, Serum Cholesterol, and Death from Coronary Heart Disease: The Western Electric Study', *New England Journal of Medicine* 304(2): 65–70, 1981, and the Honolulu Heart Study was published as 'Ten-year Incidence of Coronary Heart Disease in the Honolulu Heart Program', *American Journal of Epidemiology* 119(5): 653–66, 1984. The 2001 systematic review was published as 'Dietary Fat Intake and Prevention of Cardiovascular Disease: Systematic Review', *British Medical Journal* 322: 757, 2001, DOI: 10.1136/bmj.322.7289.757, and the 2005 Swedish study was 'Dietary Fat Intake and Early Mortality Patterns: Data from The Malmö Diet and Cancer Study', *Journal of Internal Medicine* 258)(2): 153–65, 2005.

The power of marketing The US food-availability data comes from the truly excellent databases maintained by the US Department of Agriculture's Economic Research Service. Their website is ers.usda.gov. ABARES is the Australian equivalent but provides much less historical data: daff.gov.au/abares/publications. Many of the Australian numbers cited here come from 'Commodities Consumed in Italy, Greece and Other Mediterranean Countries Compared with Australia in 1960s & 1990s', *Asia Pacific Journal of Clinical Nutrition* 2003: 12 (1): 23–29.

9. Polyunsaturated fats cause heart disease – and cholesterol doesn't

What are plant sterols? The recent studies suggesting a link between heart disease and the use of plant sterols are set out in 'Controversial Role of Plant Sterol Esters in the Management of Hypercholesterolaemia', *European Heart Journal* 30: 404–409, 2009, DOI: 10.1093/eurheartj/ehn580.

The truth about cholesterol The 2011 study that found folks with low blood cholesterol die earlier is 'Prognostic Significance of Serum Cholesterol, Lathosterol, and Sitosterol in Old Age: A 17-year Population Study', *Annals of Medicine* 43(4): 292–301, 2011, DOI: 10.3109/07853890.2010.546363.

LDL cholesterol and heart disease The 1999 study by the University of California was published as 'A Very-low-fat Diet is not Associated with

Improved Lipoprotein Profiles in Men with a Predominance of Large, Low-density Lipoproteins', *American Journal of Clinical Nutrition* 69(3): 411–18, 1999, and the 2010 Queensland study is 'Dairy Consumption and Patterns of Mortality of Australian Adults', *European Journal of Clinical Nutrition* 64: 569–77, 2010, DOI: 10.1038/ejcn.2010.45. The 2007 schoolchildren study is 'Fructose Intake is a Predictor of LDL Particle Size in Overweight School-children', *American Journal of Clinical Nutrition* 86(4): 1174–78, 2007. The study showing that Pattern A particles are less prone to oxidation is 'Susceptibility of Small, Dense, Low-density Lipoproteins to Oxidative Modification in Subjects with the Atherogenic Lipoprotein Phenotype, Pattern B', *American Journal of Medicine* 94(4): 350–56, 1993.

Are eggs really bad for you? The two major egg trials are written up in 'A Prospective Study of Egg Consumption and Risk of Cardiovascular Disease in Men and Women', *JAMA* 281(15): 1387–94, 1999, DOI: 10.1001/jama.281.15.1387, and the 2006 review showing that egg consumption converts you to Pattern A is 'Dietary Cholesterol Provided by Eggs and Plasma Lipoproteins in Healthy Populations', *Current Opinion in Clinical Nutrition and Metabolic Care* 9(1): 8–12, 2006.

Oxidised LDL and heart disease The study that shows oxidised LDL was a better predictor of heart disease is 'Circulating Oxidized LDL Is a Useful Marker for Identifying Patients With Coronary Artery Disease', *Arteriosclerosis, Thrombosis, and Vascular Biology* 21: 844–48, 2001, DOI: 10.1161/01.ATV.21.5.844.

Fructose and oxidation of LDL The major 2010 study is 'Caloric Sweetener Consumption and Dyslipidemia Among US Adults', *JAMA* 303(15): 1490–97, 2010, DOI: 10.1001/jama.2010.449.

The case for and against statins The 2007 review of statin trials was published as 'Are Lipid-lowering Guidelines Evidence-based?', *Lancet* 369(9557): 168–69, 2007, and the 2011 Cochrane review is 'Statins for the Primary Prevention of Cardiovascular Disease', *Cochrane Database of Systematic Reviews*, issue 1, article number CD004816, 2011, DOI: 10.1002/14651858.CD004816.pub4.

10. Polyunsaturated fats cause cancer

The London Hospital Study was published as 'Corn Oil in Treatment of Ischaemic Heart Disease', *British Medical Journal* 1(5449): 1531–33, 1965, and the Veterans Trial as 'Incidence of Cancer in Men on a Diet High in Polyunsaturated Fat', *Lancet* 1(7697): 464–47, 1971. A review of the 'Israeli paradox' appears in 'Diet and Disease – the Israeli Paradox: Possible Dangers of a High Omega-6 Polyunsaturated Fatty Acid Diet', *Israel Journal of Medical Sciences* 32(11): 1134–43, 1996. The rat studies on mammary cancer are summarised in 'Dietary Polyunsaturated Fat versus Saturated Fat in Relation to Mammary Carcinogenesis', *Lipids* 14(2): 155–58, DOI: 10.1007/BF02533866, and the 1997 study suggesting breast milk high in polyunsaturated fats encourages cancer in female offspring is 'A Maternal Diet High in *n*-6 Polyunsaturated Fats Alters Mammary Gland Development, Puberty Onset, and Breast Cancer Risk among Female Rat Offspring', *PNAS* 94(17): 9372–77, 1997. The 1996 Karolinska study is 'A Prospective Study of Association of Monounsaturated Fat and Other Types of Fat with Risk of Breast Cancer', *Archives of Internal Medicine* 158: 41–45, 1998.

Melanoma   A fairly recent examination of the association between outdoor work and melanoma appears in 'Cancer Surveillance Series: Changing Patterns of Cutaneous Malignant Melanoma Mortality Rates Among Whites in the United States', *Journal of the National Cancer Institute* 92(10): 811–18, 2000, DOI: 10.1093/jnci/92.10.811.

Polyunsaturated fats and melanoma   A summary of Dr Mackie's work appears in 'Melanoma and Dietary Lipids', *Nutrition and Cancer* 9(4): 219–26, 1987, DOI: 10.1080/01635588709513930.

How might polyunsaturated fats cause cancer?   The UK kidney transplant surgeons reported on their study in 'Immunosuppression with Polyunsaturated Fatty Acids in Renal Transplantation', *Transplantation* 24(4): 263–67, 1977. The study that reported on the high levels of polyunsaturated fat being stored by the folks in Israel is 'Adipose Tissue, *n*-6 Fatty Acids and Acute Myocardial Infarction in a Population Consuming a Diet High in Polyunsaturated Fatty Acids', *American Journal of Clinical Nutrition* 77(4): 796–802, 2003.

DNA damage and cancer   The 2011 study that takes a detailed look at the DNA of cancer cells is 'The Genomic Complexity of Primary Human Prostate Cancer', *Nature* 470: 214–20, 2011, DOI: 10.1038/nature09744.

Do anti-oxidant supplements work?   The 1994 trial of beta-carotene and vitamin E is the Alpha-Tocopherol, Beta-Carotene Cancer Prevention Study, which has its own website at atbcstudy.cancer.gov. The subsequent trial of vitamin A and beta-carotene is reported in 'Effects of a Combination of Beta-carotene and Vitamin A on Lung Cancer and Cardiovascular Disease', *New England Journal of Medicine* 334(18): 1150–55, 1996.

PART 3: A PRACTICAL GUIDE TO AVOIDING SUGAR AND POLYUNSATURATED FATS

12. Cutting out polyunsaturated fats (specifically seed oils)

If you're interested in what our diet looked like before industrialisation, and in particular the ratio of the various fats, then you could do worse than read 'Paleolithic Nutrition: A Consideration of its Nature and Current Implications', *New England Journal of Medicine* 312(5): 283–89, 1985.

Epilogue The quote from the Australian Heart Foundation is at heart foundation.org.au/healthy-eating/food-and-nutrition-facts/Pages/ carbohydrate-sugars.aspx. And in the *Medical Journal of Australia* (see mja. com.au/public/issues/194_06_210311/rob10104_fm.html#0_i1095900), it says: 'Although out of step with popular opinion, added sugar is not a criterion. This is because existing levels of evidence indicate that there is no direct causal relationship between added sugar and coronary heart disease, diabetes or obesity (with the possible exception of sugar-sweetened beverages).' It recommends seed oils in preference to animal fats on its website and elsewhere. The quote from the Dietitians Association of Australia is at daa.asn.au/for-the-media/ hot-topics-in-nutrition/sugar-and-obesity. On its website it also says (see daa. asn.au/for-the-public/smart-eating-for-you/nutrition-a-z/unsaturated-fats): 'Unsaturated fats are considered the "healthy" fats and are encouraged as part of a healthy diet. These fats help reduce heart disease, lower cholesterol levels and have other health benefits when they replace saturated fats in the diet.' A summary of how seed oils are regarded by the Australian Heart Foundation, the Dietitians Association of Australia, the CSIRO and the Federal Government's *Dietary Guidelines for Australians* is at spreadthefacts.com.au/expert-advice/ leading-australia-organisations.html, a website run by Goodman Fielder, the makers of Meadow Lea margarine.

Acknowledgements

I've put my wife, Lizzie, through quite a bit of change these last few years. When we decided we were no longer going to knowingly feed our children (or us) fructose, little did we appreciate how much work that would create for her. Suddenly almost all food in the middle aisles of the supermarket was off limits.

Practically, that meant that just about anything you would feed a kid has to be made from scratch. Biscuits, ice-cream and cakes all needed to be made (every single weekend) for school lunches, desserts and afternoon snacks. Fructose-free sweets were rare treats and only able to be obtained from distant and obscure shops. And there was the constant lottery as to whether the local supermarket had decided to stock dextrose at all. Multiply this by the need to do this for six growing kids (the two teenagers of which are known to eat small planets as an afternoon snack) and you had quite a workload.

When I began to understand exactly how bad seed oils were, Lizzie and I decided they had to be removed from our family's diet

258

as well. Once again, it was an easy decision for me. There was no benefit that would outweigh the insidious danger of consuming large quantities of seed oil. But it added enormously to Lizzie's load. Suddenly we had to make our own fish and chips. We had to ditch the last remaining commercial snacks we'd allowed the kids (Barbecue Shapes and chips), we had to make our own mayo from scratch, and we had to seriously contemplate making our own bread (still a bridge too far). Fun it ain't.

So for Lizzie's undying belief in my ability to interpret the science and our kids' persistence with (and even enjoyment of) what is increasingly a very olde worlde diet, I am unbelievably grateful.

Quite a few people in the media have time and again stood up and made sure that my message went out without qualification. Greg Cary from Brisbane's 4BC has been a stalwart supporter who has a talent for coaxing opponents of the no-sugar message into having little chats with me on air. And Steve Austin at the ABC has also been a huge champion of the sugar-free message. Even if I'm dull as ditchwater, Steve just keeps getting me back on the radio. I'm greatly indebted to both Greg and Steve for their persistence and determination, not to mention the weekly 'pointy-end' media training.

When your message is that people should not eat sugar, you're pitching directly against the interests of most of the processed-food industry and much of the commercial media (who depend on their advertising dollars). Many journalists have managed to persuade nervous producers and editors that getting the truth about sugar out there is just too important. I'm pretty certain this hasn't been a career-enhancing move for most of them (and for that reason I won't name them), but they know who they are and to them, on behalf of us all, I express the deepest of thanks. To those folks, the bad news is that this book targets the remainder of the processed-food industry – are you ready for this?

As always, my father-in-law, Tony Morton, has applied his extensive medical training to the raw drafts of this manuscript. He has once again been a knowledgeable sounding board as I struggled with stitching together the big picture. Having him look over my shoulder has been a crucial sanity check for me.

My friend and 'agent' Frank Stranges continued to effortlessly take care of the business stuff (I think that's the correct technical term for what he does). And that certainly takes a load off my mind.

Ingrid Ohlsson, Lou Ryan and Julie Gibbs at Penguin have been great champions of the idea that a lawyer has something important to say about nutrition, and I'm very grateful for their enthusiasm and support. Ingrid in particular has nursed (and pushed) this book from the day we first discussed it over a sugar-free lunch two years ago. Her passion for getting an important message out there was a very great motivator that made sure the book was delivered.

Nicola Young went above and beyond her editorial brief. Of course she fixed the constant barrage of split infinitives, overused brackets and just plain ordinary English. But she did much more than that. She applied her PhD brain to the facts and the evidence. She didn't just bang the words into shape, she made sure the evidence I cited actually said what I said it did. This book takes on a veritable herd of sacred cows, and in that context it is reassuring indeed to be in the hands of an editor who really knows her science stuff.

Index

A1c (HbA1c) test 118
abdominal fat 111
Abrahams, Charlie 235
Activia 84
advanced glycation end-product (AGE) 118–19, 175
agave syrup 104
alcohol 211–13
alpha-linoleic acid 221–2
Alzheimer's 119
anaemia 79
anaemia of pregnancy 67–9
animal fats 131–2, 140–1
Anitschkow, Nikolai 134–5
anti-cholesterol hysteria 180
anti-oxidants
    action 173
    in margarines 171, 173
    oxidative stress 173, 193, 194
    supplements 69, 195–6
    tocopherols 69
    variety in body 196
appetite-control hormones 105–9
appetite-control system 104–110
Apple Jacks 213–14
apple juice 206
apple sauce 214
Archer Daniels Midland foods 241
ariboflavinosis 51
arteries 132–3, 176–8

aspirin 183
AstraZeneca 181
atherosclerosis 133–5, 176–8
Atkins Diet 32, 34
Australia
    avoiding fat and heart disease 144–5, 149–50
    canola consumption 159
    deaths from heart disease 162–3
    Dietary Guidelines 41, 142–3, 144–5
    expenditure on weight loss 21–2
    fats and oils consumption 159
    nutrition policy 18
    'overweight' population 21
    spending on vitamin supplements 50
    use of statins 181
    weight-loss industry 21–2
Australia's Own Organic soy milk 209
Australian Heart Foundation 145, 162, 187
    advice on high blood cholesterol 142, 143
    recommended fat consumption 175
    'Tick' 227, 242
avocado 220

baked goods 228
Balance Bar 84
Balfour, Margaret 67
balsamic vinegar 216, 217
barbecue relish 215
barbecue sauce 214
bariatric (weight-loss) surgery 39–40
beef 149–50, 228–9
beer 211
Bellamy's toddler formula 210
beriberi 51, 53–4, 55, 61–2
beta-carotene 71, 195–6
Biggest Loser 17, 18, 28
birth defects see spina bifida
biscuits 204, 227–8
blindness 119
blood cholesterol 65, 137, 185–8, 190
blood glucose 36
    see also glycemic index (GI)
blood pressure 88–9, 137
Blue Band (food brand) 84
body fat, calories in 14
Bodytrim diet 32
bone mass 87, 88
Bonsoy soy milk 209
breads 96, 228
    what you can eat 232
breakfast
    what to avoid 237
    what you can eat 231

breakfast cereals 204, 213–14, 228
breast cancer 101, 121, 123, 187–8
breast milk 157
brewer's yeast 57–8, 67–8, 94
'brown fat' *see* glycogen
brown sauce 214
bulk minerals 85, 86–92
Bunge foods 241
butter 141, 151, 233
butyric acid 124

Cadbury chocolates 241
Cade, Dr Robert 90–1
Caesar dressing 217
calcium 65–6, 86, 87
   supplements 87
calorie
   Calorie (kilocalories) 12
   per kilogram of body fat 14
   what is it? 12
calorie consumption
   caused by weight gain 107–8
   daily calorie intake 13–14, 106
   daily requirements 23
   maintaining ideal 14–16, 19–20
   restricting 16–18
calorie content legislation 18
calorie counting 12–20
calorie labelling 18–19
cancer 101
   damage to DNA 193–5
   and folate 79–80
   and fructose 119–21
   and polyunsaturated fats 185–95
   and statins 183
   and vitamins 70–3
cane sugar 210, 211
canola oil 158–9, 190, 226, 227
Capri Sun drinks 84
carbohydrates 22, 23, 85
cardiovascular disease *see* heart disease
Cargill foods 241
carotenes 62
Castelli, Dr William 147
CCK (appetite hormone) 105, 106
cell membranes
   and polyunsaturated fats 192–3
   structure 130
Cheerios 83
cheese spread 219

childhood obesity 44–5
chips (potato) 225–6
chlorine 86
cholesterol 163, 239
   absorption and plant sterols 164–5
   and atherosclerosis 133–5
   in cell membranes 130
   dietary sources 166, 170–1, 178
   and fat 132
   feedback system 133, 166
   lowering 168
   made in body 63, 133, 166, 178–9
   restricting consumption of 166
   role 161, 165, 166–7
   statins for 164, 168, 178–84, 240
   see also HDL cholesterol; LDL cholesterol
cholesterol-free foods 180
chromium 93, 94–5, 97
chronic disease and fructose 117–19
chutneys 215
cigarettes and heart disease 137
Coca-Cola company 83, 91, 113, 115, 241
   drink 206, 211
coconut oil 141
coenzyme Q10 183
coffee 211
coffee-flavoured powder 211
Coffee-Mate 211
coleslaw, pre-made 216
collagen 60, 119
condiments 204, 214–15
confectionery *see* sweets
copper 92
   deficiency 95–6
corn oil trials 185–6
corn relish 215
cottonseed oil 152–4
cow's milk 210
cracker biscuits 227
Crestor 181
Crisco 153–4
crisps 227
Cytellin 164

daily calorie intake 13–14, 106
dairy products, what you can eat 232
Danone foods 84
dementia 79, 111, 112–13, 119
desserts 205
dextrose (glucose) 204–5

diabetes 101
   caused by fat 132, 157
   glycation end-product 118
   and low-GI (fructose-based) diet 38
   and statins 183, 184
   type 2 111, 112–13, 117, 119
diastolic blood pressure 88–9
diet industry 22
diet shakes 30–1, 211
diet soft drinks 206–7
Dietary Goals for the United States 1977 88, 142, 143, 144, 149
Dietary Guidelines for Australians 41, 131, 142–3, 144–5, 171, 178
Dietitians Association of Australia 242
diets 239
   CSIRO Total Wellbeing low-carb 32
   Dr Atkins' Diet Revolution 32
   Dukan low-carb 33
   Enter the Zone low-carb 32
   high-fat diets in history 233–7
   Paleo low-carb 32
   South Beach low-carb 32
   Sweet Poison Quit Plan 4, 202–3, 205, 206–7
   Thyroid low-carb 32
   why they don't work 6–7, 11–20, 22
   and willpower 39, 199
dinner
   what to avoid 238
   what you can eat 232
DNA damage and cancer 193–5
drinks
   artificially sweetened 206–7
   what to avoid 238
   what you can drink 232

eggs 170–1, 233
Eijkman, Christiaan 53–4
Eli Lilly 164
Endo, Akiro 179
energy drinks 207–8
energy reduction 17–18
energy-balance equation 11–12
epilepsy, diet for 234–6
Essensis 84
essential fatty acids 221–2
exercise and weight loss 1, 101, 239
   benefits 48
   drinking water 92
   theory 42–6

theory debunked 46–8
time expended on 41–2, 48
why it won't work 6, 7
working up an appetite
   48, 49

fast food calorie labels 18
fat 85
   and appetite control 13,
      105, 106
   body's requirements 233
   and cholesterol 132
   energy per gram 12, 23
   and energy storage 23
   and heart disease 132–5,
      138–9, 140–1
   high-fat diets in history
      233–7
   and hormones 129
   not worrying about 233–8
   storing 128
fat radical 172
fatty acids 221–2
   and cell membranes 130
   how they work 127–30
   long-chain 130
   omega-3 to omega-6 ratio
      223–4, 226
   oxidation 126, 171–5
   short-chain 128, 130
   and temperature 126–7
   trans fats 156–8
   as triglycerides 127, 128–9
   what are they? 123–7
   see also lipoproteins;
      monounsaturated fatty
      acids; polyunsaturated
      fatty acids
fish oil supplements 223
fish sauce 214
fizzy drinks 206, 207
flavoured coffee powder 211
flavoured coffee syrups 211
flavoured milk 204, 207
flaxseed oil supplements 223
Flora margarine 152
folate (folic acid) 66–70, 72,
   77–80
food groups 22–3
food pyramid 34
Framingham Heart Study
   146–7, 148
free radicals 172, 192–3
French dressing 216, 217
French paradox 187
fried foods 228
fries 14
fructose (fruit sugar)
   and appetite regulation
      121–2
   avoiding 102, 200–1, 203–4

and cancer 119–21
converted to fat 105, 106,
   111, 169, 200
and copper deficiency 95–6
diseases linked to 117–21,
   200
GI-lowering capability 37–8
and glucose uptake 91
and high blood sugar
   111–12
and insulin resistance 118
and iodine deficiency 95–6
and LDL oxidation 175–6
and leptin 129
low-fructose processed foods
   204–20
sources 104
as sweetener 38
and uric acid production
   89, 114–15
fruit, what you can eat 232, 233
fruit chutney 215
fruit conserves 219
Fruit Fix snack bar 242
fruit jams 219
fruit juice concentrate 218
fruit juice extract 218
Fruit Loops 214
fruit oils 6
functional foods 83–4
Funk, Kazimierz 54–5

galactose 104, 210
Gatorade 83, 90–1
General Mills foods 83, 241
gherkin relish 215
ghrelin (appetite hormone) 106
Glaceau Vitaminwater 83
glucagon 33
glucose 91, 104, 105, 118,
   204–5, 210
glycation 117–18
glycemic index (GI) 36–8
   see also low-GI diet
glycogen 34
glycosylation 117
Gobstoppers 205
goitrogens 96
Goldberger, Dr Joseph 56–8
gout 115–16
grape juice 211
Groovy Candy Rolls 205
Groovy Lollipops 205
gut bacteria 69–70

HDL ('good') cholesterol 157,
   166–7, 168
health industry 41–2
heart disease 101, 102
   Ancel Keys's work 136,
      137–42, 146

Australian death rate 162–3
cause 163
detection and options 162
and fat 132–5, 138–9,
   140–1
and homocysteine 74–5
and LDL 168–71, 173–4,
   175
prevention 163
risk factors 111, 137–9, 163
and saturated fat 132–5,
   139, 140–1, 145–51
and statins 182
and sugar 175–6
vitamins for 74–6
VITATOPS trial 75
high blood pressure 89, 116
high blood sugar 110–13
high-fat diets in history 233–7
hoi sin sauce 214
homocysteine 74–5
honey 104, 204, 219
Honolulu Heart Study 147–8
Hopkins, Sir Frederick 54
hormones
   appetite control 105–9
   and cholesterol 165
   and fat management 129
   and obesity 108–10
   role 107
   thyroid 95, 96
hunger 17–18, 19
hunger signal 33–4
hydrogenation 153, 154,
   157–8, 160
hypertension 142

ice-cream 204, 205–6
immune system impairment
   52
Indigenous Australians 113,
   115
insulin 105
   and appetite control 106
   and GI rating of food 38
   resistance 94–5, 110, 111,
      118
   sensitivity 94
inulin 26
iodine 92, 208–9
   deficiency 95–6
iodised salt 95
iron 92
   deficiency 93–4, 95
Israel data on polyunsaturated
   fats 186–7, 192
Israeli paradox 187
Italian dressing 217

Jalna fruit yoghurts 218
jams 219

Jenny Craig 21
  does it work? 27–9
  fat-elimination diet 24,
    26–7
joule 12
juices 204, 207, 218

Kashi cereals 84
Kellogg's 84, 213–14, 241
ketchup 214
ketoacidosis 236
ketogenic diet 234, 235–7
ketones 234
Keys, Ancel 55, 135, 156,
  158, 234
  K-rations 136
  and 'Mediterranean diet'
    141–3, 155
  research 16, 18, 136,
    137–42, 145, 146
KFC 151, 224
kidney disease 89–90, 113–15
kilocalories (Calorie) 12
kilojoule (kJ) 12
Kraft foods 84, 241
K-rations 136

labels 226–7
lactose 104
lactose intolerance 208, 210
laksa sauce 215
lap-band surgery 39–40
LDL cholesterol 164, 167
  and atherosclerotic lesions
    176–8
  'bad' 168
  and heart disease 168–71,
    173–4, 175
  oxidation 171–6
  Pattern A and B particles
    168–70, 192
lemon juice dressing 217
leptin (appetite hormone) 105,
  106, 129
leukaemia 79
linoleic acid 126, 191, 221–2
linseed oil supplements 223
lipids 172
Lipitor 180–1
lipoproteins 127, 167
liqueurs 212
Lite n' Easy 24, 26–7
liver 69, 166, 178–9
London Hospital Study 185–6
lovastatin 179
low-calorie versus low-GI
  diet 37
  see also low-fat/low-calorie
    diets
low-carb diets 22
  Atkins Diet 32, 34

do they work? 33–4, 38–9
hard to stick with 36–7
hunger signals 33–4
popular diets 32–3
'special foods' 32
versus low-fat diet 33–5
low-density lipoproteins 167
low-fat/low-calorie diets 22,
  23–7
  cutting 100 calories per
    day 9
  do they work? 27–9
  hunger all the time 33–4
  and sexual desire 165
  versus low-carb diet 33–5
low-fructose processed foods
  204–5
low-GI diet 36–7
  dangers of fructose 37–8
  versus low-calorie diet 37
Lucozade Original 208
lunch
  what to avoid 237
  what you can eat 232

McDonald's 14, 19, 150–1,
  159, 224
Mackie, Dr Bruce 189–90, 192
macrophages 174, 177
magnesium 86, 87
Malmö Diet and Cancer Study
  148
maltose 211
manganese 92
Mann, Traci 38–9
maple syrup 104
margarine 126, 150, 201,
  227, 233
  anti-oxidants in 171, 173
  development of 151–2
  vitamin D fortification 53
Marmite 68, 69
Mayer, Jean 42–4
Mayo Clinic 48, 234
mayonnaise 215–16
meal replacement diets 22,
  29–31
meat
  protein in 23
  and uric acid 113–14
  vitamins in 50, 70
  what you can eat 232, 233
'Mediterranean diet' 141–3,
  155
Mège-Mouriès, Hippolyte
  151–2
melanin 188, 194–5
melanoma 64, 66, 101, 188,
  188–90
Mellanby, Sir Edward 62–3
mental retardation 95

Merck & Co. 179, 180, 181
metabolism and weight loss
  17–18
Mevacor 179, 180
mevastatin 179
Mike & Jack sweets 205
milk 206, 229, 233
  enzyme-treated 210
  flavoured 204, 207
  low-fat 169
  vitamin D in 65–6
milk substitutes 208–10
mineral water 206
minerals
  bulk 85, 86–92
  supplements 97
  trace 85, 92–6, 97
mixer sauces 228
mixers (drinks) 212
molybdenum 93
monounsaturated fatty acids
  124–5, 130, 157–8, 188,
  221
Monte Carlo biscuit 14, 46
muesli 217
muesli bars 204, 217
multivitamins 76–7, 93–4
mustard 215
myelin 165
myelination 95

Nesquik 84
Nestlé foods 26, 84, 205, 211,
  240–1, 242
neural tube defects 52, 70, 72,
  78, 96
Newburgh, Louis 45–6
night blindness 52
nitric oxide 89, 116, 176
Normann, Wilhelm 153
nut oils 6
Nutella 38
nuts 229, 230, 233
  what you can eat 232

oat cereals 204
obesity 101
  and chronic disease 110–21
  and hormone dysfunction
    108–10
Odwalla juices 83
oils
  combination of fatty acids
    126
  labelling 226–7
  relative stability 172
oleic acid 125
olive oil 125, 141, 158–9
olive-oil dressing 217
omega-3 fatty acids 222–4, 226
omega-6 fatty acids 222–4

'organic sugar' 210
Organic Toddler Milk 210
osteoporosis 76, 80, 87
'oven-fry' goods 228
oxidation 126171–5
oxidative stress 173, 193, 194

palm oil 224–5
pancreas 104, 119–21
Pauling, Linus 73–4, 81
Paul's foods 210
peanut butter 219
pellagra 51, 55–8, 67
PepsiCo foods 83, 91, 241
peripheral temperature 18
pesto 215
Pfizer 180, 181
phosphorus 86, 87
phytosterols see plant sterols
plant sterols 163–5
polycystic ovary disease 111
polyunsaturated fats 125–6
    and cancer 185–95
    cutting out 221–30
    and heart disease 162
    industry growth 152–6
    measuring intake 192
    not manufactured by body
        126, 176, 221–2
    and oxidation 171, 192–3
    US consumption 156
polyunsaturated seed oils 102,
    150, 155–6, 199–201
porridge 204, 214
port 212
potassium 85, 86, 90
powdered drinks 210–11
Powerade 91
PowerBar 84
Praise mayonnaise 216
pregnancy
    anaemia of pregnancy 67–9
    iron deficiency 93–4
    neural tube defects 52, 70,
        72, 78, 96
    thyroid hormones 95
processed foods 86, 201
    low-fructose 204–20
Procter & Gamble 153–4
prostate cancer 121, 123
Protein Power low-carb diet
    32
proteins 23, 85, 93
Pukara Estate mayo 216

Quaker Oats 83

ranch dressing 217
raw oats 228
reactive oxygen species 192–3
Red Rock Deli 227

relishes 215
retinoid therapy 80
rice 53–4
rice milk 209
rickets 53, 62–3, 65–6
rock salt 95

salad dressings 215–17
salsa 215
salt 239
    daily needs 86–7
    dangers 87, 88, 89, 141
    iodised 95
salt tablets 90–1
salt-hypertension hypothesis
    142
sandwich toppings 232
Sanitarium
    So Good soy milk 209
    Up & Go range 228
saturated fat 124, 130, 161,
    221
    and heart disease 132–5,
        139, 140–1, 145–51
    in red meat 149–50
sauces 204, 214–15
    mixers 228
Scandinavian Simvastatin
    Survival Study 180, 182
scar tissue 165
scurvy 52, 58–61
seed oils 104, 126, 224, 243
    avoiding 6, 200–1, 221–31
    cottonseed oil 152–4
    Crisco 153–4
    hydrogenation 153, 154,
        157–8
    market growth 155–6, 199
    other uses 160
    polyunsaturated fat content
        155–6
    soybean oil 154–5, 157–8,
        159
    success of industry 155–6,
        160–1, 199
    tocopherols in 69
    vitamin E source 53
seeds 229, 230
selenium 93
sex drive and weight loss 16
shakes 30–1, 211
short-chain fatty acids 128,
    130
simple sugars 104
simvastatin 180
Slim-fast 84
smoking 137
snack bars 217
snacks
    what to avoid 238
    what you can eat 232

So Natural soy milk 209
soda water 206
sodium 86, 90
soft drink 204
    health effects 106, 113,
        115–16, 120–1
    low-fructose 206–8
sorbitol 206
soy milk 86, 96, 208–10
soy sauce 215
Soya King soy milk 209
soybean oil 154–5, 157–8, 159
Special K cereal 84
spina bifida 52, 70, 72, 77–8,
    80
sports drinks 90–2, 207–8
spreads 204, 218–20
    what to avoid 238
    what you can eat 232
starvation studies
    Biggest Loser participants 17,
        18, 28
    Minnesota trial 16, 18
statin drugs 240
    and cancer 183
    and cholesterol 164, 168,
        178–84
    creation and marketing
        179–81
    and diabetes 183, 184
    for and against 182–4
    and heart disease 182
    trials 182–4
steak sauce 214
stearic acid 191
sucrose 104, 210
sugar 89, 94–5, 96, 102
    and appetite control 109–10
    avoiding 122, 200–1, 203–4
    conversion to fat 103,
        121–2
    and heart disease 175–6
    'organic' 210
    simple sugars 104
    see also fructose
Sugar Crisp 213
Sugar Smacks 213
sunflower oil 229
sunflower seeds 229
sunscreen 63, 64, 65
supplements
    calcium 87
    fish oil 223
    flaxseed oil 223
    industry 6, 55
    linseed oil 223
    see also anti-oxidants;
        minerals; vitamin
        supplements
sweating 90
sweet chilli sauce 214

INDEX

Sweet Poison 4
Sweet Poison Quit Plan 4,
   202–3, 205, 206–7
sweet sherry 212
sweets 204
   low-fructose 205–6
systolic blood pressure 88–9

Tabasco sauce 215
taco sauce 215
tartare sauce 214
tea 211
thousand island dressing 216
thyroid gland 95–6
thyroid hormones 95, 96
tocopherols 69
toddler formulas 210, 211
tomato chutney 215
tomato relish 215
tomato sauce 214
trace minerals 85, 92–6, 97
trans fats 156–8
triglycerides 105, 127, 128–9
type 2 diabetes 111, 112–13,
   117, 119

Unilever foods 84, 152, 241
United States
   beef and chicken
      consumption 149–50
   cholesterol treatment
      guidelines 181
   exercise-participation 42
   national dietary guidelines
      88, 142, 143, 144, 149
   overweight population 21
unsaturated animal fats 140–1
Up & Go range 228
uric acid 60, 89–90, 113–16,
   119

vegans 62, 70, 86, 97
Vegemite 68, 219
vegetable oils 6, 141, 150
vegetable-based shortening
   cottonseed oil 152–4
   Crisco 153–4
   hydrogenation process 153,
      157
   soybean oil 154–5
vegetables 233
   what you can eat 232
vegetarians 62, 93, 94

very low-calorie diets 28,
   29–30, 34–5
Veterans Trial 186, 190
vinegar 216, 217
vitamins
   as cancer cure 70–3
   discovery 53–70
   fat-soluble 51, 52–3
   food sources 50, 51–2
   for heart disease 74–6
   overconsumption 51
   water-soluble 51–2
vitamin A (retinol) 52, 61–3,
   65, 70, 71, 80–1
vitamin B group
   B1 (thiamine) 51, 53–5
   B2 (riboflavin) 51
   B3 (niacin) 51, 55–8
   B5 (pantothenic acid) 52
   B6 (pyridoxine) 52, 74
   B7 (biotin) 52
   B9 (folate/folic acid) 52,
      66–8, 72
   B12 (cobalamin) 52, 74,
      79
   as cancer treatment 71–2
   discovery 55–8
   and heart disease 74–5
vitamin C (ascorbic acid) 52,
   58–61, 70, 72, 73–4, 75–6
vitamin D 53, 62–6, 70, 72–3,
   87, 165
vitamin E 53, 69, 72–3, 75–6,
   195–6
vitamin K 53, 69, 76
vitamin supplements
   adding to food 82–4
   Australian spending on 50
   dangers 77–80, 80, 81
   multivitamins 76–7, 93–4
   need for 77, 81, 87
   self-medicating 74, 81
   why they don't work 81–2
'vitamin waters' 207–8
vitamin-deficiency diseases 51,
   52, 53–69
Vitasoy soy milk 209
VITATOPS trial 75

Warner-Lambert 180, 181
water
   and exercise 92
   unflavoured 206

water retention 88
weight gain
   and age 14
   calculating 14–15
   and calorie consumption
      107–8
   and hormone dysfunction
      108–10
   over time 14–15
weight loss
   Australian expenditure on
      21–2
   common themes 22
   and metabolism 17–18
   and sex drive 16
   and willpower 39
weight-loss industry 21–2
weight-loss methods
   DIY 21–2
   low-carb 22, 32–8
   low-fat/low calorie 22,
      23–9, 33–5, 165
   meal-replacers 22, 29–31
   surgery 39–40
Weight Watchers 21, 24–9
Western Electric Company
   Study (US) 147, 148
wholegrain cereals 94
Wills, Lucy 66–9
wine 211–12
women
   bone mass 88
   daily calorie needs 23
   in pregnancy 52, 70, 72,
      78, 96
   statins of no benefit 182–3
Woodyatt, Rollin 234
Woolworths Home Brand bread
   228
Worcestershire sauce 214

xerophthalmia 61–2

Yakult foods 84
yoghurt 83, 201, 204,
   217–18
Yoplait yoghurts 83

zinc 85, 92, 93–4
Zocor 180
Zymil 210